Let's Eat!

A Clinical Guide to the Management of Complex Pediatric Feeding and Swallowing Disorders

Angela Mansolillo MA, CCC-SLP, BCS-S

All identifying information, including names and other details, has been changed to protect the privacy of individuals. This book is not a substitute for continuing education or professional supervision, or for seeking advice from a trained professional. The author and publisher disclaim responsibility for any adverse effects arising from the application of the information contained herein.

Published by
PESI Publishing
PESI, Inc.
3839 White Ave
Eau Claire, WI 54703

Cover: Amy Rubenzer
Editing: Jenessa Jackson, PhD
Layout: Amy Rubenzer & Bookmasters

ISBN: 9781683734130

Printed in the United States of America

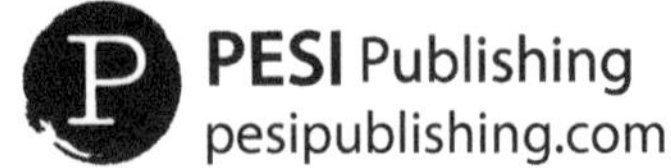

Dedication

For my clients, who struggle daily with what comes so easily to the rest of us. I'm in awe of your courage and determination. And for your parents and caregivers who only ever want what's best for you—and who don't stop working until they get it. It is my privilege to work with you and for you.

For my own parents and siblings, who taught me the importance of family and food...and how the two go together!

And for James and Jim (whose first response was "You're writing a book?"), with thanks for your patience and your love, and of course, for the laughter. My life is so much better with you in it!

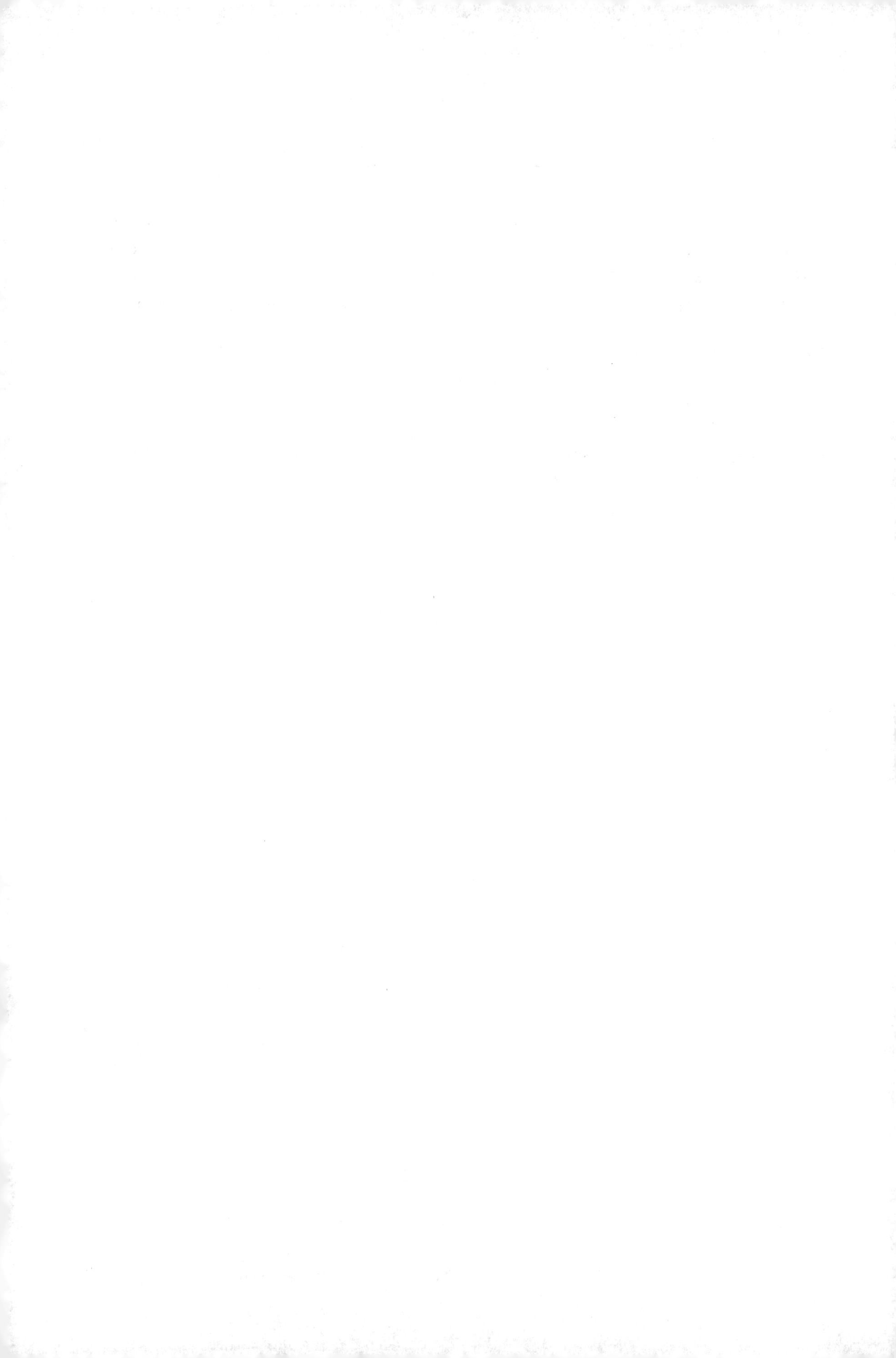

About the Author

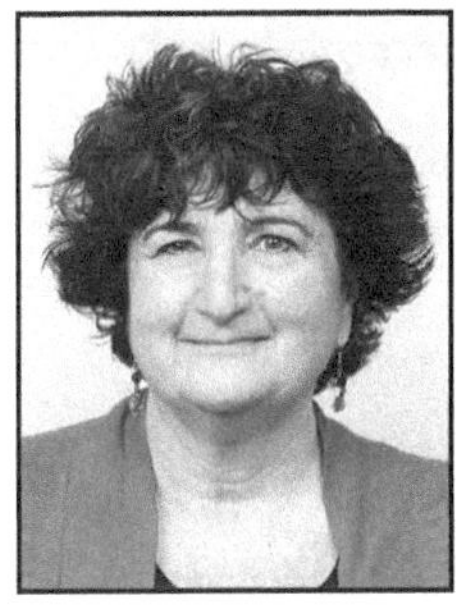

Angela Mansolillo, MA, CCC-SLP, BCS-S,

is a speech-language pathologist and Board Certified Specialist in Swallowing and Swallowing Disorders with over 21 years of experience. She is a clinical supervisor and adjunct faculty member at Elms College Department of Communication Sciences and Disorders. She has worked in a variety of clinical settings, provided numerous regional and national presentations, and served as guest lecturer at several colleges and universities.

Ms. Mansolillo received her Bachelor of Arts degree in communication from Rhode Island College and earned her Master of Arts in speech-language pathology from the University of Connecticut.

Table of Contents

Introduction

"I didn't know anybody did this kind of work." I can't tell you how many times I've heard people say this to me over the course of my career. Parents who had struggled for months or even years trying to feed their children. Physicians who had no resources for their patients who were aspirating or choking, or who just wouldn't or couldn't eat. Families who had been told by their school or early intervention teams that "we're just not trained to do that." Parents frustrated by well-meaning family members advising them to "just wait, she'll eat when she's hungry." Clearly, there is a continued lack of awareness in the medical community, and in the general public, regarding the options for remediation of feeding and swallowing difficulties in children.

Those of us who work with children with feeding and swallowing difficulties know we're in the minority among dysphagia clinicians and among clinicians in general. A 2019 survey by the American Speech-Language-Hearing Association (ASHA) revealed that 40 percent of speech pathologists employed in health care settings work with pediatric clients, but children with feeding and swallowing disorders make up only 15 percent of those clients. Moreover, only 10 percent of school clinicians report treating feeding and swallowing disorders, and for those who do, the average number of children on their caseloads is an underwhelming four clients (ASHA, 2020)!

Unfortunately, many university programs put a lower priority on pediatric feeding and swallowing issues in their coursework, and clinicians just do not get the training they need to feel comfortable working with children in these areas. Therefore, this book is designed to assist clinicians in assessing feeding and swallowing dysfunction in pediatric populations, as well as (and more importantly) to determine the underlying cause (or causes) of that dysfunction. Given that a great deal of the available dysphagia research focuses on adults—and it is more difficult to complete research with children for sure—you'll find that while I utilized the available pediatric research, I have also borrowed from the adult research base as well.

Chapters 1 and 2 provide information about typical feeding and swallowing development and describe tools to assess dysfunction in these areas with a focus on identifying potential etiologies. Once you have an understanding of those causative factors, the subsequent etiology-based chapters in this book are intended to help you develop treatment plans that are impairment-focused. As my Introduction to Special Education professor told our class over and over (and over) again, "You've got to know the cause!"

Finally, in the appendices you will find a variety of sample feeding and swallowing treatment plans, as well as tips to help you develop measurable treatment goals and conduct feeding and swallowing therapy via telehealth.

I am a speech-language pathologist by training and a rehabilitation professional at heart. It is clear to me that our clients are best served when the members of their teams collaborate with each other. I have learned a tremendous amount from the occupational therapists, physical therapists, registered dieticians, nurses, physicians, and other team members I have had the good fortune to work with in my career. Therefore, this book is not written for clinicians of any particular discipline but for any of us who work with the broad spectrum of babies and children with feeding and swallowing difficulties.

Let's Eat! is a reflection of my core beliefs as a clinician. I believe parents and caregivers are essential partners in our work to remediate feeding and swallowing disorders. To facilitate that partnership, you'll find parent and caregiver information, tips, and handouts throughout the book. I also believe eating is a social activity, as well as a physiological one, and have tried to include as many potential eating partners and environments as possible throughout these chapters. And I believe eating should be enjoyable, comfortable, and—yes—even fun. Ultimately, my hope is this book will help increase awareness of what is possible for infants and children with feeding and swallowing disorders...so *let's eat!*

1

Understanding Normal Feeding and Swallowing

What exactly is "normal"? When it comes to feeding and swallowing, normal encompasses a wide range of behaviors, motor movements, physiological and neurological responses, and sensory reactions. Given that eating develops in conjunction with postural stability, motor skills, cognition, language, respiration, and neurological development, this chapter will not only discuss how and when children acquire feeding and swallowing skills but also place those skills in the context of overall infant and child development.

WHAT IS A PEDIATRIC FEEDING DISORDER?

Defining a pediatric feeding or swallowing disorder is not as easy as it would seem. Speech-language pathologists use terms like *oral phase dysphagia* or *pharyngeal dysphagia*. Occupational therapists may make a distinction between sensory and motor disorders. There are multiple terms in the literature, including *picky eater*, *restricted food repertoire*, *failure to thrive*, and *infantile anorexia*. Recently, avoidant/restrictive food intake disorder (ARFID) was added as a diagnosis to the fifth edition of the *Diagnostic and Statistical Manual of Mental Disorders* (DSM-5®; APA, 2013) to describe the feeding difficulties that often accompany autism spectrum and other sensory-based disorders. However, none of these diagnoses truly captures the complexity and diversity of children with feeding and swallowing disorders.

In 2019, an interdisciplinary group of pediatric experts convened and developed a new diagnosis called pediatric feeding disorder, which is characterized by the following criteria: "impaired oral intake that is not age-appropriate, and is associated with medical, nutritional, feeding skill, and/or psychosocial dysfunction" (Goday et al., 2019). According to this definition, pediatric feeding disorder can be acute (< 3 months in duration) or chronic

(≥ 3 months in duration), must have been present daily for at least two weeks, and is diagnosed only in the *absence* of body image disturbance. According to this framework, pediatric feeding disorder is associated with one or more of the following dysfunctions:

1. **Medical dysfunction** (e.g., aspiration, respiratory infection, respiratory disease)
2. **Nutritional dysfunction** (e.g., malnutrition, specific nutrient deficiency, reliance on enteral feeding)
3. **Feeding skill dysfunction** (e.g., need for texture modification, need for modified feeding position or equipment, use of feeding strategies)
4. **Psychosocial dysfunction** (e.g., active or passive food avoidance, disrupted caregiver-child relationship associated with feeding, disrupted social functioning within a feeding context)

Describing the disorder, while important, is not always helpful in treatment planning though. **Effective treatment planning is dependent on our ability to identify the underlying cause or causes of the feeding disorder.** This diagnosis of pediatric feeding disorder, while well described, is not a true diagnosis. No disorder occurs in a vacuum. Something (or more than one something) is causing that disorder, and until we know what those causes are, we will be unable to build a viable treatment plan.

So what are some of the potential causes of pediatric feeding disorder? They include impaired respiration, gastrointestinal (GI) dysfunction, motor impairments, sensory disorders, and pharyngeal swallow dysfunction. Our clients have neurological disorders, genetic syndromes and congenital issues, developmental delays, and acquired disorders. They are a widely heterogeneous group of children. If our treatment plans do not take into consideration all of their underlying issues, the plans will fail.

"What about behaviors?" you're asking. Yes, maladaptive behaviors have the potential to restrict repertoire, limit oral intake, and cause a great deal of frustration for parents and therapists. They certainly must be addressed, and we will discuss how to do that in chapter 6. We must be careful, however, not to attribute too much causation to maladaptive behaviors. More often than not, these problematic behaviors are the *result* of the feeding or swallowing disorder rather than the cause. We will not be successful in addressing the behaviors unless and until we have first identified and addressed the underlying issues.

WHAT DOES "NORMAL" LOOK LIKE?

Before we begin to think about diagnosing and treating feeding and swallowing disorders, we first need an understanding of normal development. Obviously, babies and children develop individually, and what's considered "normal" encompasses a wide range of feeding and swallowing characteristics. However, it is important to discuss "typical" development as we move forward.

Prenatal Development

It is beyond the scope of this chapter to discuss embryology and fetal development in detail, but there are a few important things to know about prenatal development:

- **The respiratory system and GI system develop from the same embryonic structure.** The tracheoesophageal septum is formed during weeks 4–5 of fetal development and divides the foregut into ventral and dorsal sections. The ventral portion develops into the larynx, trachea, bronchi, and lungs, while the dorsal portion develops into the esophagus. It is difficult to deny a relationship between breathing, swallowing, and digestion given that these systems all develop from the same structure!
- **Pharyngeal swallow generally appears between 10–14 weeks of gestation.** The role of fetal swallowing as it relates to amniotic fluid volume regulation is not clear. There appear to be a number of factors at work, but this regulation does appear, at least in part, to depend on fetal swallow frequency (Beall et al., 2007). In addition, these early swallows provide the fetus with its first exposure to tastes.
- **Suckling begins between 18–24 weeks of gestation.** Mouthing and tongue movements are often present earlier in fetal development, but true suckling begins in the second trimester. Suckling rates increase as fetal growth continues (Miller et al., 2003).
- **The alveolar period of lung development does not begin until *after* the infant is born.** The alveolar spaces in the lungs are the end points of bronchial division, and it is here that the gas exchange critical to respiration occurs. Prior to birth, at or around 32 weeks of gestation, less mature saccules form. Mature alveoli do not develop until after birth—when the infant is breathing air. Surfactant production, too, takes place very near term. *Surfactant* is a foamy fluid in the lungs that keeps the alveolar spaces open and available for gas exchange. Without it, the alveoli collapse and respiratory distress results. Clearly,

these developmental considerations have implications for infants with pharyngeal dysphagia, as aspiration into a still-developing lung will have different consequences than aspiration into a more fully developed lung. These consequences will be explored further in subsequent chapters.

Infant Anatomy

There are some important differences between infant and child anatomy to consider. In the infant, the presence of suckling pads narrows the oral cavity and facilitates bolus transfer. The tongue takes up proportionately more space in the mouth in the infant than in the child or adult. It has a higher resting position, typically resting against the hard palate. The soft palate sits lower in the pharynx and, in fact, approaches the vallecular spaces. The vocal tract is shorter, making the nasopharynx and oropharynx indistinguishable from each other. The hyoid bone is not completely ossified, which makes it more difficult to see on radiographic swallow studies. It has a higher resting position in infants, just below the mandible.

The larynx also sits higher in the pharynx in infancy—typically between the first and third cervical vertebrae—and is in a more protected position under the tongue base. The epiglottis is also higher and in some infants actually touches the velum. It is narrower and has a vertical orientation. During the swallow, the larynx only moves anteriorly, not vertically, and we do not see epiglottic retroversion over the larynx. Given the position of the airway and epiglottis, the forward tilt of the arytenoids is sufficient to contact the base of the epiglottis and provide airway protection. These differences allow for coordination of sucking, swallowing, and breathing, as well as airway protection, in a reclined position (Arvedson et al., 2020).

Preterm infants, of course, are likely to have even more dramatic differences in anatomy and physiology. Oral and pharyngeal structures are smaller, and oral reflexes, such as suckling and rooting, are often absent. Suckling pads may not have developed, and overall muscle tone is low.

As the infant moves into childhood, the vocal tract gets longer, and a more pronounced oropharynx forms. The tongue base, larynx, and epiglottis descend, and the soft palate and epiglottis separate. Suckling pads in the oral cavity are slowly absorbed. This increases the space in the oral cavity and facilitates development of the more sophisticated lingual movements required to manage solid food boluses.

Developing Feeding and Swallowing Skills

Feeding and swallowing milestones occur in concert with one another and in conjunction with a variety of other developmental processes, including the development of postural stability, respiration, cognition and attention, GI functions, and motor skills. All of these systems interact with one another as the infant moves from suckling at the breast or bottle to managing a wide variety of food types using a wide variety of utensils.

The Role of Postural Stability

Infants maintain overall body flexion during the first month after birth, and this flexion facilitates oral feeding by supporting early suckling and maintaining the pharyngeal airway. As the infant begins to move against gravity and bear weight (in the prone position initially), movements become more purposeful and controlled. With increasing trunk, shoulder, head, and neck support, oral movements become more sophisticated (Massery, 1991).

Postural stability continues to be linked with motor function as the child develops into their toddler and school-age years. Increasing stability in the core—with resulting increases in head and neck stability—facilitates increased jaw stability, which is critical for bolus manipulation and mastication. A stable jaw also provides support for the tongue and lip movements required for bolus management, chewing, and utensil use.

Pharyngeal Swallow and Airway Protection

The act of swallowing serves two distinct but related purposes: (1) transfer of food and liquid from the oral cavity to the stomach and (2) closure and protection of the airway. Initially, suckle and swallow are tightly coupled as the infant utilizes the suckle to initiate a swallow. By six months of age, infants can produce a swallow without an initiating a suckle or suck, which represents the beginning of voluntary control over the swallow response. The following steps are involved in the swallow response:

- Bolus transit begins in the oral cavity and varies depending on the bolus type and utensil. In infancy, liquid boluses are extracted from a nipple via suckle or suck and are propelled via tongue movement posteriorly to the pharynx. Pureed boluses are cleared from a spoon via active upper lip movement and similarly propelled backward. As texture increases, more lingual manipulation is required, including lateralization of the food to the teeth for chewing. Once well-chewed, the food is transferred back to midline and propelled to the pharynx.

That posterior propulsion is accomplished via tongue-to-palate contact. The soft palate elevates, and the posterior pharyngeal wall contracts to close the nasal airway. Pharyngeal constrictor muscles contract in sequence in a stripping wave that—together with tongue-base propulsion—moves the food or liquid through the pharynx. The upper esophageal sphincter opens to facilitate transfer of the food and liquid through the pharynx into the esophagus.

- Airway closure, too, is a multistep process. As the food and liquid enter the pharynx, respiration pauses. Hyoid elevation elevates the larynx under the tongue base. (This is less pronounced in infants as the larynx sits higher in the pharynx at rest in infancy.) The upward and forward movement of the larynx facilitates closure of the laryngeal valve, which is further accomplished by medialization of the aryepiglottic folds and the vocal folds. Contact between the underside of the epiglottis and the arytenoids provides additional airway closure.
- Infant oral and pharyngeal anatomy, as discussed earlier, is different from that of the child or adult. Consequently, there are differences in swallow physiology as well. Given the position of the tongue, the posterior tongue does not elevate to initiate a swallow as it does in children and adults. Instead, the suckle itself initiates the swallow response and the driving forces produced by the tongue pull the hyolaryngeal complex forward, and the upper esophageal sphincter opens to allow bolus transit into the esophagus. Given that there is little to no epiglottic movement in infants, the valleculae act as "holding" sites for the bolus until the airway closure is complete.

These systems work well to propel food and liquid and to protect the airway, but material does enter the airway at times. We have all had the experience of aspirating, particularly when we are talking or laughing while eating and drinking. When that occurs, protective mechanisms are triggered to clear the airway of the aspirated material. In infants, this is largely accomplished via prolonged breathing cessation in conjunction with additional swallows. Over the first few months of life, a cough response develops, and cough is then utilized to either keep material out of the airway or get aspirated material out of the airway.

Breathing and Swallow Coordination

As noted, breathing pauses during the swallow to facilitate airway protection. Breathing and swallowing, therefore, must be well coordinated during feeding and swallowing. Typically, the swallow interrupts the exhalation portion of the breathing cycle, resulting in an exhale-swallow-exhale pattern. In infancy, however, it is not uncommon to see an inhale-swallow-exhale pattern, which converts to an exhale-swallow-exhale pattern within the first few months of life. This post-swallow exhalation serves several purposes, including clearance of any post-swallow residue, facilitation of laryngeal elevation and closure, and promotion of esophageal clearance (Lau, 2016).

Suck-swallow-breathe coordination is critical in infants. The three systems are interdependent and function together to facilitate effective feeding, state regulation, and sleep patterning. Rhythmic sucking triggers a regular swallow response and efficient respiratory control.

Infants are preferential nasal breathers. For anatomical reasons (e.g., smaller oral cavities, presence of suckling pads), it is easier to move air through the nasal cavities than through the oral cavity in infancy. During feeding, infants will produce suckle bursts—two to three suckles, followed by a swallow and a breath.

Lung Functions

Our lungs have a number of different responsibilities, and an understanding of these functions is critical to our understanding of breathing-swallow coordination and aspiration management. These functions include respiration, ventilation, and pulmonary clearance.

Respiration: The exchange of oxygen and carbon dioxide between the atmosphere and the cells of the body

Respiration occurs because gas molecules will always move from high pressure to low pressure. We bring oxygen into our lungs via an inhalation, and pressure increases. The oxygen then diffuses through the alveolar spaces into the bloodstream. Red blood cells attach themselves to the oxygen molecules and transport them to the cells throughout our body. Oxygen enters the cells, and a conversion to energy occurs. The byproduct of that conversion is carbon dioxide (CO_2). As CO_2 levels increase within the cell, pressure increases, and CO_2 diffuses through the cell membrane into the venous bloodstream, where it is carried back to the lungs. Rising levels of CO_2 trigger the next inhalation, and the process begins again.

Because swallowing requires breathing cessation, it places significant demands on the respiratory system. Your client's respiratory rate is one way to assess their response to those demands. Assessment of the respiratory rate at rest and during feeding and swallowing trials can provide valuable insights into airway protection.

Ventilation: The mechanical movement of air through the respiratory system

Ventilation is accomplished via movements of the respiratory muscles and the expansion of the ribcage. Muscles responsible for ventilation, particularly the intercostal muscles, are also critical to the development and maintenance of core stability (Massery, 1991). Therefore, not only are children with impaired core stability going to have postural instability, but they are also likely to present with respiratory insufficiencies. It will be important to pay close attention to breathing-swallow coordination in these clients.

Pulmonary clearance: Removal of foreign material from the airways

Everybody aspirates. But not everybody develops aspiration pneumonia. That's because most of us have intact pulmonary clearance mechanisms that are designed to keep material out of the airways or remove material from the airway. There are three pulmonary clearance mechanisms:

1. **Cough:** We use cough in two ways: (1) to keep material from entering the airway and (2) to remove material from the airway. Cough is often *not* present at birth, as the cough reflex develops over the first few months of life. Cough is variable but does have predictable components. It requires inhalation, adduction of the vocal folds, and forceful exhalation to clear the airway.

2. **Mucociliary clearance:** Within the body of the lungs, the bronchi and bronchioles are lined with hair-like structures called cilia. The cilia are coated with mucus and move in rhythmic waves in the lung fluid. That beat-like movement essentially brushes the foreign matter up toward the main bronchi, where it can be coughed out.

3. **Cellular clearance:** Cellular clearance mechanisms are mediated by the immune system, which provides white blood cells to scavenge through

the lungs and absorb foreign matter in a process called phagocytosis. Foreign matter—food, liquid, and even bacteria to a certain extent—are phagocytized or absorbed and eliminated from the lungs.

If these pulmonary clearance mechanisms fail and the foreign matter is not cleared, illness is likely.

Aspiration and Illness

The fact that we have the ability to clear foreign matter from our lungs raises a couple of questions: "Who gets sick from aspiration?" and "How much aspiration is too much aspiration?" Let's examine those questions one at a time:

1. **Who gets sick from aspiration?**

   In order to answer this question, we have to think about what we know about this child's potential for using those pulmonary clearance mechanisms we just talked about:

   a. **Cough:** Children who can use cough to clear their airway are at lower risk for the development of pneumonia or other aspiration-related respiratory illnesses. Therefore, silent aspiration—that which occurs without a protective airway response like coughing—is more likely to result in illness. We also have to consider the strength and efficacy of the cough. Children with a weak cough response (due to weak respiratory musculature, weak core musculature, or impaired lung function) are at higher risk of illness as well.

   b. **Mucociliary clearance:** Impairments in cilia motility clearly result in reduced mucociliary clearance, but how do we know which children have impaired cilia motility? We can't see the cilia and internal workings of the lungs during our assessment, but we can use what we know about the child's history and current status to provide us with some insights into ciliary function. Is this a child who had a period of ventilator dependence or dependence on high-flow nasal cannula in infancy? We know that those high-pressure interventions, necessary as they may be, have the potential to damage cilia. We also know that when we are dehydrated, our cilia don't move very efficiently, and clearance is reduced. Remember, cilia move in lung fluid, so if lung fluid is reduced, as it is during periods of dehydration, cilia motility is reduced. Unlike high-pressure ventilatory supports, though, dehydration does not damage cilia. Once we rehydrate, cilia motility returns to its baseline level of functioning.

c. **Cellular clearance:** Remember that cellular clearance is a function of the immune system. That means that babies and children who are immunocompromised are going to be less likely to mount an effective cellular clearance response. Ask yourself, then, what are the medical conditions and comorbidities that are impacting this child's immune system functioning? These are limiting factors with regard to pulmonary clearance as well. Is this a child who is currently fighting an infection? A child who is frail and underweight? A child who has a number of comorbidities? The more demands on the immune system, the less able the child will be to protect themself from aspiration-related illnesses. We also need to think about the child's nutritional status. Our immune systems are fueled by good nutrition, so the child who is underweight and undernourished is likely to be immunocompromised and, in turn, unable to perform efficient pulmonary clearance.

2. **How much aspiration is too much aspiration?**

Perhaps the most important thing to consider as we assess the potential consequences of aspiration is the aspirate itself. What do we know about the material that entered the lung? Was the aspirated material highly acidic? Aspiration of acidic reflux can be very dangerous in the lung and often results in illness. As feeding therapists, we of course pay a great deal of attention to prandial aspiration, so what was the child eating or drinking when the aspiration happened? Foods and liquids are cleared differently depending on their molecular makeup, weight, and bacterial content. Proteins and fat-based foods are typically harder to clear than water-based foods like fruits. Therefore, phagocytosis is more efficient when the aspirate is water-based. Heavier solid foods are also harder to clear than liquids because mucociliary clearance can be more efficient with aspirates that weigh less. And the more bacteria contained in whatever is aspirated, the harder it will be to clear, and the greater the risk.

Age and lung development are additional considerations as we assess our client's potential to manage aspiration. Remember what we learned about lung development, specifically alveolar development? Babies have little alveolar space compared to older children and adults. Pneumonia is an infection in alveolar spaces, so babies are less likely to develop pneumonia as a result of aspiration. Instead, aspiration in infancy is more likely to result in inflammation, which can have unfortunate consequences in a still-developing lung. Chronic aspiration that leads to chronic inflammation in the first six months of life can result in permanent lung damage—changes in the lung at a cellular level—that put the infant at risk of greater susceptibility to lung infections and disease. Clearly, we must be very vigilant about aspiration management with our youngest clients.

So how does an aspiration-related illness occur? In order for illness to develop, three things have to happen:

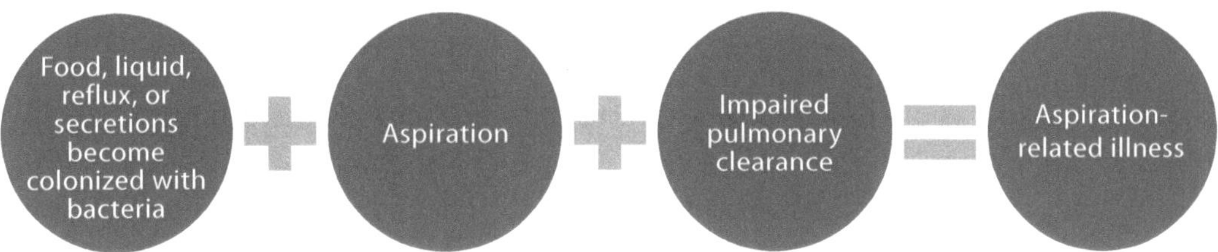

Which of the children on *your* caseload are at high risk of illness? Let's examine those steps one at a time to find out:

1. Whatever is aspirated—be it food, liquids, saliva, or reflux—becomes colonized with bacteria. How does that happen? The oral cavity is a common source of bacteria. Children with **dental decay** or **poor oral hygiene** are more likely to have high bacterial counts in their mouths and are therefore more likely to aspirate larger amounts of bacteria. Tubes—feeding tubes, ventilator tubing, or tracheostomy tubes—are also common sources of bacteria, which puts **tube-dependent children** at higher risk of illness.

2. The colonized material is then aspirated. Children known to have **dysphagia** are clearly at high risk for illness. So are children with **reflux disease** who may be experiencing reflux that enters the airway.

3. The aspirated material is not cleared from the lungs effectively. That means that children with an **impaired cough response**, children who are **dehydrated or undernourished**, children with **impaired cilia integrity**, and **immunocompromised** children will be at higher risk.

We can use this framework, then, to identify the children on our caseload who are at higher risk of aspiration-related illnesses as we conduct our assessment.

Suckle to Suck

During nippling, two different patterns of liquid extraction may be observed. The less mature *suckle* is present in utero and is the first pattern utilized for early oral feeding. During suckling, the lips are quite loose around the nipple, and it is the tongue that cups the nipple to provide the seal. Suckling is characterized by front-to-back tongue movements that extract the liquid from the nipple by creating negative pressure. During breastfeeding, the cupped tongue pulls the nipple into the oral cavity as far as the juncture of the hard and soft palates. During bottle-feeding, the nipple remains in place and the infant only needs to compress it. The fatty suckling pads that are present in the cheeks in infancy help stabilize the tongue during feeding.

Beginning around six months of age, a more mature *suck* pattern emerges. Lip closure around the nipple increases and creates the seal required to extract liquid. Suckling pads become smaller, and cheek muscles become more developed. This, combined with the increasing size of the oral cavity, help increase tongue mobility. The tongue begins to move in an up-down plane during nippling as the tip and sides of the tongue move up to the palate and then depress in sequence. Vertical jaw movements continue during sucking but with reduced width of excursion.

Both suckling and sucking are efficient patterns of liquid extraction, but delayed transition to sucking may have consequences for transition to other utensils and bolus types. If the suckle pattern persists, the tongue is essentially "locked in" to the anterior-posterior movement pattern, which delays the development of lateralization and, in turn, delays the transition to textured boluses. In addition, if the lip seal continues to be loose, spoon clearing and transition to cup and straw drinking may be impacted.

Breast versus Bottle

Recently, ultrasound studies examining the mechanics of breastfeeding have brought current models of milk extraction into question (Douglas & Geddes, 2018). In particular, this research has found that current structural models of sucking are flawed because they miscalculate the primary mechanism of milk transfer. To understand, let's look at the mechanics of breastfeeding in more detail.

Both breastfeeding and bottle-feeding require suck-swallow-breathe coordination, adequate seal to extract liquid from the nipple, and intact oral control. However, bottle-feeding requires more cheek and lip movement than breastfeeding. The infant only needs to compress the nipple for liquid extraction, as the nipple on the bottle stays in place without any work on the part of the infant. Bottle-feeding typically results in shorter pauses between suckle bursts. Bolus sizes are often larger with bottle-feeding than with breastfeeding, which appears to be because the breastfeeding infant has more control over the flow rate and bolus size.

Breastfeeding infants have long been thought to extract liquid from the breast via suction, but recent ultrasound studies have demonstrated that the vertical movements of the jaw and tongue create an intraoral vacuum that draws milk from the breast (Douglas & Geddes, 2018). The process begins as the lips and face come into contact with the breast tissue, triggering a mouth-opening response as the infant takes the breast tissue (the nipple and surrounding tissue) into the mouth. As the jaw and tongue (functioning as a single unit) drop, the oral cavity enlarges, and the intraoral vacuum increases, which draws milk from the breast into the mouth. The jaw and tongue then return to midline, and the breast tissue is compressed (during which time no additional milk flows), the milk passes over the back of the tongue, and a swallow response is triggered.

Tethered Oral Tissue: What's Normal?

Recently, tongue- and lip-ties have been getting a great deal of attention from pediatricians, lactation consultants, and feeding therapists. Unfortunately, we are just beginning to understand what normal oral tissues look like and how they function. The *lingual frenulum*, which is the structure implicated in tongue-ties, connects the tongue to the floor of the mouth. It is a normal structure, and the vast majority of us have one. It is sometimes described as a band or cord, but a recent cadaver study revealed that the frenulum is, in fact, a discrete structure. It is actually a fold in the layer of connective tissue that forms the floor of the mouth (Mills et al., 2019). Labial (or lip) ties are sometimes thought to limit breastfeeding by limiting lip flange and subsequent latch. All infants have some degree of attachment of the upper lip to the maxilla, however. This tissue may serve as a place holder of sorts for the incisors. Therefore, instead of focusing our attention on the tissue as we make recommendations for or against revision, we can better serve our clients by placing our focus on its function.

Teeth

There is a great deal of variability in both the timing and the sequence of teeth eruptions. Typically, the central incisors come in first, followed by the lateral incisors, first molars, canines, and second molars, but it is not uncommon to see individual differences. Deciduous (or baby) teeth begin to erupt as early as 6 months, and eruptions continue thereafter. Permanent teeth emerge between ages 6 and 12, and third molars (wisdom teeth) erupt during the teenage years or later. Before, during, and immediately after eruptions of deciduous teeth, "teething" behaviors often occur. Irritability, drooling, biting, or sucking behaviors increase and may interfere with appetite and intake.

Taste and Smell

Taste and smell are important to many aspects of feeding, including food acceptance, regulation of intake volume, and perhaps initiation of the swallow response as well. Prenatal exposure to taste occurs as the fetus swallows amniotic fluid, meaning that the mother's diet during pregnancy has the potential to impact food repertoire in the toddler years (Mennella et al., 2001). Breastfeeding has a similar impact as it, too, provides early exposure to a wide variety of tastes (Forestell, 2017; Mennella, 1995).

Infants appear to be born with the ability to perceive sweet and sour tastes, as studies have found that they reject sour-tasting liquids and accept those that are sweet tasting. They are typically more indifferent to bitter and salty tastes until approximately four months of age (Mennella, 1995).

Appetite Regulation

Infants typically indicate hunger by crying and rooting, while they indicate satiety by discontinuing suckling, slowing the suckling pace, or pulling away from the nipple. By 3 to 4 months of age, infants will open their mouth in anticipation of a nipple or spoon and may also reach for the nipple or spoon to indicate hunger and interest in eating. As foods are introduced, the child will adjust their breastmilk or formula intake accordingly and will indicate satiety by turning away from the nipple or spoon. By 9 to 10 months, the child can point to food to indicate interest, and by 12 months and beyond they will use language to communicate both their desire to eat or drink and their specific choices and preferences.

Gastrointestinal Development

Postnatally, our GI system does not necessarily develop on a schedule but develops, at least in part, based on intake. We begin with nutritionally complete and easily digestible foods (breastmilk, infant formula) and progress to the digestion of larger volumes of food and more complex foods. This process, called *gut priming*, facilitates formation of the gastric microbiome, which is critical, not only for digestion, but for immune system function and perhaps for cognitive and neurological development as well (Clarke et al., 2014).

There are trillions of microbes, and thousands of species of microbes, in the human body, mostly in the gut. In fact, the microbes in our bodies outnumber human cells by a ratio of 10 to 1! Your microbiome is specific to you and contains inherited microbes, as well as those you've acquired through environmental exposures and diet.

The human microbiome develops in three phases: the developmental phase (3 to 14 months), the transitional phase (15 to 30 months), and the stable phase (31 to 64 months; Stewart et al., 2018). The fetal microbiome does not appear to be very diverse, but significant colonization occurs during the birthing process. Many factors—such as feeding method (breastmilk versus formula), skin-to-skin contact, environmental exposures, and medications—have an impact on colonization in the first few months of life. A diverse, balanced microbiome protects us from pathogens, facilitates digestion, metabolizes toxins and medications, and promotes immune system functioning.

Respiratory-Gastrointestinal Connections

The respiratory system and GI systems interact in a number of ways, including via pressure and energy. These two systems are adjacent to each other in the chest cavity and exert pressure on each other. For example, it is not uncommon to see respiratory changes, such as increased work of breathing or increased respiratory rate, in babies and children who are experiencing reflux. That's because the expanded stomach and esophagus displace the lungs—in other words, put pressure on the lungs—and work of breathing increases as a result. The opposite relationship is also one to consider. Whenever the lung is overinflated—for example, during exertion or respiratory distress—it puts pressure on the esophagus and stomach. As a result of this pressure, reflux potentially increases.

A second way the two systems interact is through the body's energy requirements. At any given time, our bodies have a finite amount of energy available to us. Healthy babies and children have plenty of energy—in fact, they have reserves of energy—but our more fragile clients may not have sufficient energy to meet their daily demands. When energy is insufficient, organ systems in the body compete for available energy, and in any competition, breathing always wins! Where does that energy come from? One place is the digestive system. As work of breathing increases, and energy is pulled to the respiratory system, digestion slows. And as digestion slows, reflux often increases.

Much of the respiratory and GI system is innervated by the vagal nerve, so any disruption in the vagal response could potentially cause problems in both systems. What does this mean for our work with babies and children with feeding and swallowing problems? If we are working with a child with respiratory issues, they are likely to have GI issues as well. And if we are working with a client with reflux disease or other GI issues, respiration is likely to be affected too.

Finally, there are also a number of allergens that impact the entire aerodigestive tract, which I will discuss in chapter 3.

Nutrition and Growth

Most babies lose 5 to 10 percent of their birth weight after birth but begin gaining and growing by two weeks of age. A typical baby will double their birth weight by four to six months of age and will triple it by the time they are one year old.

Between birth and three months, babies are expected to:

- Gain approximately 1 ounce per day
- Grow ½ to 1 inch per week

Between three and six months, babies are expected to:

- Gain 5 to 7 ounces per week
- Grow approximately 1 inch per week

Between six months and twelve months, babies are expected to:

- Gain 3 to 5 ounces per week
- Grow approximately ⅜ inch per month

Between one year and five years, children are expected to:

- Gain approximately 5 pounds per year
- Grow 1 to 2 inches per year

Between five years and puberty, children are expected to:

- Gain approximately 5 pounds per year, with weight gain increasing as puberty approaches
- Grow approximately 2 inches per year

Of course, these developmental growth averages are dependent on a child receiving good nutrition. What does good nutrition look like? *Infants* generally meet all of their nutritional needs via breastmilk or infant formula. Breastfed babies will feed more frequently than formula-fed babies because formula takes longer to digest. Newborns can be expected to feed every two to four hours and, as they grow, will go longer between feedings. In most babies, breastmilk or formula will provide all of the nutritional requirements, but some breastfed babies may need zinc, vitamin D, or iron supplementation.

The benefits of breastfeeding are well-known and well-documented but bear repeating. Breastfeeding provides immune system protections—both immediately and over the lifetime—and it also facilitates the development of a healthy microbiome, improves gastric emptying, and provides infants with exposure to a wide variety of tastes.

Solid foods are introduced gradually, starting at six months. Most commonly, iron-fortified baby cereal is the first food, followed by pureed fruits and vegetables.

Toddlers are sometimes in a precarious position when it comes to nutrition. Children at this age are transitioning from receiving all of their nutrition from a single source (breastmilk or formula) to meeting their needs from a variety of food sources. This can result in nutritional deficiencies, particularly with regard to calcium, vitamin D, and iron. Fiber intake is often reduced as well.

As *children* reach the age of 3 and beyond, they make more independent food choices and, as a result, sometimes have limitations in their diet. Variety should be encouraged, and children should have a number of different proteins, grains, fruits, and vegetables in their diets.

Age	Caloric Requirements
Birth to 6 months	500–700 calories per day (5–8 feedings per day)
6 to 12 months	800–900 calories per day (3–4 feedings per day)
12 months to 36 months	1000 calories per day (3 meals per day and snacks)
3 years to 8 years	1200–1400 calories per day (more for active children)
9 years to 13 years	1400–1600 per day for girls (more for active children) 1600–2000 per day for boys (more for active children)

Macronutrients are substances that our bodies need in large quantities in order to function—in other words, carbohydrates, fats, protein, and water. *Micronutrients* are dietary substances that our bodies need in smaller amounts but are nonetheless critical to our health and well-being, such as various vitamins and minerals. As illustrated in the following tables, nutritional deficiencies in either of these areas can have a number of feeding-related consequences for babies and children.

Macronutrient	Signs of Deficiency
Calories	Muscle wasting, growth limitations
Protein	Impaired immune system function, muscle wasting, slow wound healing
Fat	Impaired brain development
Fluid	Constipation, dehydration

Micronutrient	Signs of Deficiency
Calcium	Impaired bone growth
Iron	Anemia, weakness, fatigue
Zinc	Poor growth, delayed wound healing, impaired taste
Vitamin D	Weak tooth enamel
Vitamin C	Dry mouth, gingival changes
Vitamin B	Glossitis, taste alteration, dysphagia, paresthesia

In children with developmental disabilities, there is evidence to suggest that periods of malnutrition in infancy and early childhood can have long-term consequences on growth and development. Further, nutritional interventions later in life may not be effective, seeing as malnutrition often progresses over time (Schwarz, 2003). Therefore, nutritional assessment should begin in infancy for clients with neurological impairments, developmental delays, or medical compromise and should occur regularly thereafter.

You can find additional information about typical growth and weight gain at the Centers for Disease Control and Prevention (CDC) website. Here you can access growth charts developed by the World Health Organization (WHO) and the CDC (https://www.cdc.gov/growthcharts), as well as BMI calculators for toddlers and older children (https://www.cdc.gov/healthyweight/bmi/calculator.html). In addition, the American Academy of Pediatrics has created a website at www.healthychildren.org that provides parents and caregivers with information about a variety of topics, including serving sizes and nutritional needs in babies and children.

Feeding and Swallowing Developmental Milestones

Infancy and childhood are busy times, with tremendous amounts of development occurring in systems that impact feeding and swallowing. The following chart summarizes maturation in feeding and swallowing skills and in some of the systems that support them.

Age/ Stage	Postural Control/Motor Development	Swallowing	Respiration	Oral Motor	Food Types
Newborn	Flexion; Feeder provides external stability; Ribs horizontally aligned; Anterior chest wall is tight secondary to flexion	Suckle pattern; Suckle/swallow ratio 1:1	Nasal breathing	Lips, tongue, and jaw function as single unit; No differentiation present	Breastmilk or infant formula
1–3 months	Head control and purposeful movements emerge; Extremity movement increases	Suckle continues; Suckle/swallow ratio 2–3:1	Nasal breathing; Suckle-swallow-breathe coordination improves	Jaw and lip movements increase	Breastmilk or infant formula
3–5 months	Head control increases; Rolling over begins; Sits supported with head control; Upper chest wall movement	Suckle continues; Suck emerges near end of this period	Tidal volume increases as a result of chest expansion and lung development; Less frequent pauses for breaths during feeding	Increased lip, jaw, and tongue differentiation; Gagging with texture is not uncommon	Breastmilk or infant formula; Purees
6 months	Sits unsupported; Transfers objects from hand to hand	Transitions to true suck; Uncoupling of suckle and swallow	Rib cage expansion results in increased tidal capacity and improved respiratory and phonatory control	Jaw and tongue differentiation; Gag reflex is less sensitive	Finger feeding begins; Mouths objects, toys, and fingers; Clears spoon with upper lip

Age/ Stage	Postural Control/Motor Development	Swallowing	Respiration	Oral Motor	Food Types
7–9 months	Crawls; Pulls to stand; Can rotate, flex, and extend while sitting	Transition to suck continues	Ongoing improvements in phonatory, respiratory control but less coordinated with introduction of cup	Vertical jaw movements	Cup drinking introduced; Manages thicker purees and soft solids
10–12 months	Stands; Walks or cruises; Ongoing chest expansion (able to move chest walls laterally, superior-inferiorly, and in A-P plane); Pincer grip emerges	True suck	Improved breathing-swallow coordination with cup	Vertical chewing pattern emerges; Rotary jaw movements emerge	Weans from nipple to cup; Manages ground/ mashed table foods
13–18 months	Independently walks; Climbs stairs	Well-timed and coordinated across bolus types	Well-coordinated across bolus and utensil types	Complete lip and tongue differentiation; Lingual lateralization	Full cup use; Straw drinking; Manages coarser, highly textured solids
18–24 months	Balance improves			Sustained bite; Rotary chew	Manges a wide variety of solid foods, including meats and raw vegetables
24 months and beyond	Jumps; Runs; Grasps and releases with precision			Graded jaw movements; Smooth lingual bolus transfer across midline; Chew continues to become more efficient	One-handed cup drinking; Fork use

2

Assessment: Getting to the Underlying Issues

ETIOLOGY MATTERS

Feeding and swallowing disorders don't just appear out of nowhere; something causes them. Identifying what that cause might be is critical not only to our overall assessment process but also to the development of an appropriate treatment plan. There are a number of potential causes—breathing, digestion, and aspiration, to name a few—and we need to be sure we design our assessment process in such a way that we can accurately recognize those causes.

It is important to realize that the initial evaluation is just the beginning of the assessment process. Initial observations can be misleading, especially because children are sometimes on their best behavior and perform better than they typically would at home. Alternatively, some children are anxious about the assessment and eat less well than they typically would in other environments. What children eat, how they eat, when they eat, and how much they eat are all likely to fluctuate depending on the setting, the people in the environment, the way they are positioned, the foods they are eating, and the utensils they are using. In other words, if you've seen one meal...you've seen one meal!

THE ASSESSMENT PROCESS

Case Review and Parent Interview

The assessment process generally begins with a thorough case history and interview of the parents or other caregivers and feeders. We gather information about the child's medical history, birth history, and current medical concerns, as well as information regarding feeding behaviors and characteristics. The following section provides more detail on the types of questions to ask in each of these areas.

Medical History Questions

- **Medications currently taking:** Look for medications that could be sedating or cause irritability, as well as medications that could cause pharyngeal dysphagia or GI issues. (See the "Medications and Feeding/Swallowing in Children" handout in this chapter for more information regarding specific medications and their effects on feeding, swallowing, and GI function.)
- **Pregnancy complications:** Ask about magnesium sulfate therapy, maternal drug use, and prenatal drug or alcohol exposure.
- **Birth history:** Determine the child's gestational age at birth, medical complications at birth, need for respiratory support, need for non-oral feeding, and length of stay in the neonatal intensive care unit (NICU) if applicable.
- **Medical diagnoses:** Does the child have any allergies, congenital syndromes or other genetic conditions, neurological conditions, seizure disorder, vocal fold dysfunction, or cardiac issues? Has the child ever undergone any surgical procedures? Has the child had pneumonia or other aspiration-related illnesses?
- **Pertinent lab results:** What does lab work tell you? Are there any nutritional deficiencies, infections, or respiratory issues that might be impacting feeding or swallowing? (See the "Lab Results: What Should the Feeding and Swallowing Therapist Know?" handout in this chapter for guidance regarding lab results as they relate to feeding and swallowing.)
- **Aspiration:** Are there concerns regarding pharyngeal dysphagia and aspiration? Do you observe any clinical signs of aspiration, such as coughing, choking, changes in breathing, or changes in vocal quality?
- **Oral health:** Does the child receive regular dental care? Are there issues around toothbrushing tolerance? Are there known oral health issues, including cavities, oral infections, tooth loss, or pain?
- **Prior testing, procedures, or surgeries:** Look for chest X-rays or CT scan results, as well as CT scans or MRIs of the head. Has any swallow testing been done? Has the child undergone any modified barium swallow (MBS) studies or flexible (fiberoptic) endoscopic evaluation of swallow (FEES) tests? (See the box on the following page for a description of X-ray and CT scan terminology.)

- **General developmental history:** Are there concerns about cognitive function? Gross motor function? Fine motor function? Speech and language?
- **State regulation:** Do the parents note frequent irritability? Lethargy? What strategies have been successful in alerting or calming the child? Does the infant or child have any self-calming strategies (e.g., sucking, mouthing)?

Guide to Chest X-Ray and CT Scan Terminology

Chest X-Ray Terminology

1. Density, opacity, infiltrate: Airspaces have been filled with foreign matter
2. Consolidation: A more diffuse opacity
3. Atelectasis: Collapse of alveoli with loss of lung volume
4. Edema: Fluid in alveolar or interstitial spaces
5. Effusion: Fluid in pleural cavity

Chest CT Scan Terminology

1. Parenchymal bands: Fibrotic tissue
2. Bronchiolectasis: Abnormal enlargement of small airways (bronchioles)
3. Bronchiectasis: Abnormal enlargement of larger airways (bronchi)
4. Bronchial wall thickening: Thickening of bronchi/bronchioles, typically associated with inflammation
5. Atelectasis: Lung collapse
6. Tree-in-bud pattern: Nodules in a branching pattern, typically associated with infection
7. Ground-glass opacities: Fluid in airspaces and thickening of tissue around alveoli; can be associated with a variety of pathologies, including infection

Respiratory History Questions

- **Known respiratory conditions:** Does the child have a history of asthma? Bronchopulmonary dysplasia? Bronchiolitis? Apnea?
- **Oxygen support:** When was (or is) it necessary? How is the oxygen provided? What is the flow rate?
- **Tracheostomy and/or mechanical ventilation:** When did this occur? Is ventilatory support required currently? Is there a speaking valve in place? How does the child manage their secretions? How often is suction required?
- **Upper respiratory infections, pneumonias:** When did the child have the infection and what type? Are there concerns regarding aspiration?
- **Respiratory changes during feeding:** Does the child exhibit coughing, choking, or a wet-hoarse voice with eating or drinking? When is this observed? Are there changes in respiratory rate or effort with eating or drinking? If so, when does this occur?

Gastrointestinal History Questions

- **Tube feeding:** How is nutrition delivered? What is the schedule? What formula is used? Is a blended diet being utilized?
- **Reflux:** Is there a history of reflux? Are there currently concerns about reflux? How often does it occur? What are the symptoms? What are the triggers?
- **Inflammatory issues:** Does the child ever complain about pain with eating or drinking? Are there concerns about reflux esophagitis or eosinophilic esophagitis (EoE)?
- **Vomiting:** Are there concerns about vomiting? How often does it occur? What appears to trigger it?
- **Stooling:** Are there concerns about constipation or diarrhea? Have the parents noted discomfort or straining with bowel movements? Is the child anxious about stooling? How often does the child move their bowels?
- **Food allergies:** Does the child have a current or past history of food or other allergies? Is there a family history of allergies? Has any allergy

testing been completed? If so, what type of testing was done, and what were the results?

- **Congenital GI issues:** Does the child have evidence of fistulas, esophageal atresia, or other intestinal issues?

Feeding History Questions

- **Weight gain and growth:** Are there concerns about growth or weight gain? Are the child's current height and weight age appropriate or diagnosis appropriate?
- **Early feeding history:** Was the infant fed via breast or bottle? Were there any difficulties? Did the child transition successfully to pureed foods? To solid foods? To cup drinking?
- **Nutrition:** Are there concerns about adequacy of intake? Variety of intake? Volume of intake? Does the child consume age-appropriate food types? Use age-appropriate utensils? Are there sufficient protein sources in the child's diet? Does the child eat fruits and vegetables? If so, which ones and how often? What are the family's patterns and habits around eating?
- **Current feeding:** What is the current feeding schedule? How much does the child consume at a typical meal? How long does a typical meal or feeding take? What foods are typically offered to the child? What foods does the child accept or refuse? What happens when the child refuses foods?
- **Food repertoire:** What are the child's preferences regarding food taste, texture, and temperature? How does the child respond to various tastes, temperatures, or textures? Does the child refuse certain foods or liquids? If so, which ones? What foods or liquids does the child dislike? If the child refuses foods, how does the parent or caregiver respond?
- **Utensil use:** What utensils does the child use? Are self-feeding skills age appropriate? Does the child refuse any utensils?
- **Positioning for feeding:** Where does the child eat? How is the child positioned or seated? Does the child remain seated throughout the meal?
- **Fluctuations in performance:** Who feeds or eats with the child? Does the child's intake fluctuate with different feeders? In different places?

Throughout the day? Throughout the meal? How long has the problem been going on? What makes it better? Worse?

- **Parental concerns:** What do the parents see as the biggest challenge? What foods would they like to add to their child's repertoire first? What approaches have they tried? What worked? What didn't work?

On the following pages, you will find several handouts and forms that can assist you in the assessment process as you gather information regarding the child's history. There are also handouts to help you better understand the effects of certain medications on feeding behaviors and to allow you to more easily interpret the child's lab results.

Parent/Caregiver Form

Feeding Behavior Questionnaire

Child's name: ______________________________

Name of person completing form: ______________________________

Relationship to child: ______________________________

Date: ______________________________

Think about your child's feeding behaviors in the last 30 days:

My child...	Frequently	Sometimes	Never
Was upset or agitated during mealtimes	☐	☐	☐
Left the table before the meal was done	☐	☐	☐
Spit out food or liquid	☐	☐	☐
Gagged during eating	☐	☐	☐
Gagged when smelling food	☐	☐	☐
Was inflexible about where, when, or what they ate	☐	☐	☐
Was unwilling to try new foods	☐	☐	☐
Ate the same foods at each meal	☐	☐	☐
Refused food based on its texture	☐	☐	☐
Refused food based on its appearance	☐	☐	☐
Refused food based on its smell	☐	☐	☐
Insisted that food was served in a particular way	☐	☐	☐
Was unable or refused to use a spoon or fork	☐	☐	☐
Was unable or refused to use a cup	☐	☐	☐
Coughed or choked	☐	☐	☐

Again, thinking about the last 30 days:

I worry that...	Frequently	Sometimes	Never
Other people are unable to help because they are afraid to feed my child	☐	☐	☐
Other people are unable to help me because my child won't eat for or with them	☐	☐	☐
My child is not well nourished	☐	☐	☐
My child does not get enough to eat or drink	☐	☐	☐
My family cannot go out to eat or make plans that involve eating or food	☐	☐	☐
My child is excluded from activities with other children because of their feeding issues	☐	☐	☐

Clinician Form

Case History

Client: ______________________ DOB/age: ______________

Food allergies: ______________________________________

Medical diagnoses: ___________________________________

Height/weight: __________ / __________

Growth/weight gain concerns: __________________________

Parent concerns: _____________________________________

____

Feeding

Tube feeds? Tube type? Formula? Schedule? _____________

____

____

Supplements: ____

____

____

Typical PO Intake

☐ Liquids ☐ Puree ☐ Textured foods ☐ Chewables/biteables

Amounts: ____

____

Self-Feeding

Utensils used:

☐ Bottle ☐ Sippy cup ☐ Open cup ☐ Spoon ☐ Fork

☐ Straw ☐ Finger feeding

How do you know when your child is hungry, thirsty, or full?

____

____

How long is a typical meal?

____

____

Positioning for Eating

Do you notice:

- ☐ Choking
- ☐ Gagging
- ☐ Labored breathing
- ☐ Drooling
- ☐ Food refusals
- ☐ Coughing
- ☐ Vomiting
- ☐ Difficulty swallowing
- ☐ Irritability with eating
- ☐ Difficulty chewing
- ☐ Changes in breathing
- ☐ Wet voice
- ☐ Biting

Comments:

____

____

Medical History

- ☐ Pneumonia/respiratory infections
- ☐ Surgical procedures
- ☐ Reflux/constipation/other GI issues
- ☐ Neurological deficits
- ☐ Ear infections
- ☐ Craniofacial issues
- ☐ Cardiovascular issues

Comments:

____

____

Food Preferences

	Likes	Dislikes
Taste	______	______
Temperatures	______	______
Textures	______	______
Utensils	______	______

Instrumental Assessment

Date of assessment: ____________________

Type of assessment conducted:

____

____

Reason for assessment:

____

____

Where was it conducted?

____

____

Results:

____

____

____

____

____

Previous/Current Interventions:

____

____

Parent Goals for Therapy:

____

____

____

____

____

Clinician Handout

Medications and Feeding/ Swallowing in Children

Medications, whether prescribed or over-the-counter, can have a profound effect on feeding and swallowing function. Use this handout to think about the medications your client is taking as well as the potential impacts you should be looking for.

Medications can impact:

- Motor function: Anticonvulsants, antipsychotics, antianxiety medications
- GI function: Antihistamines, antipsychotics, anticholinergics, bronchodilators, diuretics
- Arousal: Anticonvulsants, narcotics, muscle relaxants
- Salivation: Anticholinergics, antihistamines, antidepressants, antipsychotics
- Taste or smell: Anticholinergics, antibiotics, chemotherapy agents
- Pharyngeal swallow: Anticonvulsants, antipsychotics, antianxiety medications

Type of Medication	Examples	Purpose	Potential Impact on Feeding and Swallowing
Antianxiety medications	Buspirone (Buspar®), Clonazepam (Klonopin®)	Reduce anxiety via reduction in brain activity	• Sedation, lethargy • Altered mental status • Reduction in motor control • Altered taste • Xerostomia • GI upset
Antibiotics	Penicillin, Amoxicillin, Metronidazole (Flagyl®)	Treat infections	• Alterations in taste • Metallic taste • Loss or diminishment of smell
Anticholinergics	Doxylamine (Unisom®), Dimenhydrinate (Dramamine®), Diphenhydramine (Benadryl®)	Treat allergies, nausea, incontinence, and excess secretions	• Reduced GI motility • Vomiting • Xerostomia • Dizziness
Anticonvulsants	Phenytoin (Dilantin®), Carbamazepine (Tegretol®), Levetiracetam (Keppra®)	Used for seizure control, neuropathic pain control	• Mucosal hypersensitivities • Gingival hyperplasia • GI upset • Sedation
Antidepressants	Fluoxetine (Prozac®), Sertraline (Zoloft®), Venlafaxine (Effexor®)	Treat depression by influencing levels of neurotransmitters in the brain	• Sedation • Reduced GI motility • Dry mouth, constipation

Type of Medication	Examples	Purpose	Potential Impact on Feeding and Swallowing
Antihistamines	• H_1-antihistamines (Allergy treatment): Diphenhydramine (Benadryl), Cetirizine (Zyrtec®), Fexofenadine (Allegra®) • H_2-antihistamines (GERD treatment): Ranitidine (Zantac®), Famotidine (Pepcid®)	Control GI and allergy symptoms via opposition of histamine receptors	• Xerostomia • Dizziness, nausea • Altered mental status, sedation • Altered GI function • Irritability
Antipsychotics	• First generation (Typical): Haloperidol (Haldol®), Chlorpromazine (Thorazine®) • Second generation (Atypical): Clozapine (Clozaril®), Risperidone (Risperdal), Aripiprazole (Abilify®), Quetiapine (Seroquel®)	Control psychotic symptoms and treat bipolar disorder; Typical antipsychotics have higher risk of side effects compared to atypicals	• Dystonia • Sedation • Xerostomia • Reduced GI motility • Impaired swallow response
Appetite stimulants	Megestrol acetate (Megestrol®), Cyproheptadine (Periactin®)	Increase hunger and appetite	• Stomach upset • Constipation • Xerostomia • Drowsiness or • Irritability
Bronchodilators	Albuterol, Theophylline	Open airways by relaxing smooth muscles	• Nausea, vomiting • Irritability

Type of Medication	Examples	Purpose	Potential Impact on Feeding and Swallowing
Chemotherapy agents	Elspar®, Myleran®, Carboplatin	Treat cancer	• Xerostomia • Altered taste, smell • GI upset (nausea, vomiting, diarrhea) • Mucosal injury (oral cavity, pharynx, esophagus, GI tract) • Reduced appetite • Reduced arousal • Increased respiratory effort
Diuretics	Lasix®	Used in premature infants to reduce fluid around the heart; Used for the treatment of congestive heart failure, fluid retention	• Nausea, vomiting, constipation • Oral and/or gastric irritation
Muscle relaxants (Antispasmodics)	Baclofen, Dantrolene	Decrease muscle tone to facilitate movement and/or relieve pain	• Sedation, fatigue • Dry mouth • Dizziness
Narcotics	Morphine, Codeine, Phenobarbital (sometimes prescribed as an anticonvulsant)	Relieve pain	• Sedation, respiratory depression *or* agitation, irritability • Nausea, vomiting, constipation • Dizziness • Respiratory changes

Clinician Handout

Lab Results: What Should the Feeding and Swallowing Therapist Know?

As feeding therapists, we are *not* making medical diagnoses based on lab work. Rather, we are building a basic understanding of lab values that can help us have more informed conversations with team members; alert us to the possible presence of infection, respiratory issues, or nutritional deficiencies; and generally help round out our picture of our client. Abnormal lab values can signify a variety of different issues, particularly in medically complex clients, but this handout highlights those issues that may be feeding or swallowing related.

Lab Value	What It Measures	What It Could Mean
White blood cell (WBC) count	Provides information about immune system function	• Abnormally high numbers of WBCs typically indicate the presence of infection • Abnormally low results may indicate impaired bone marrow function or the presence of an autoimmune disorder
White cell differential	Provides information on the number of white blood cells in each category: • Neutrophils • Eosinophils • Basophils • Lymphocytes • Monocytes	Helps identify the *type* of infection: • Neutrophils increase with bacterial infections • Eosinophils increase with allergic reactions • Basophils increase with inflammation • Lymphocytes increase with viral infections • Monocytes increase with infections in general
Red blood cell (RBC) count	Provides information about the body's ability to maintain oxygenation	• Abnormally high numbers can indicate dehydration • Abnormally low results can indicate anemia, the presence of a disease process, or limited ability to maintain oxygenation
Hematocrit	Reflects the percentage of RBCs in total blood volume	• Abnormally high numbers can indicate dehydration • Abnormally low numbers can indicate anemia or reduced oxygenation
Hemoglobin	Measures the protein responsible for oxygen transport	• Abnormally high numbers can indicate dehydration or respiratory illness • Abnormally low numbers may indicate anemia or reduced oxygenation
Blood urea nitrogen (BUN)	BUN is a waste product of protein metabolism that provides insight into kidney function	• Abnormally high results can indicate dehydration or renal failure • Abnormally low numbers can indicate impairments in protein metabolism, reduced protein absorption, or nutritional compromise

Lab Value	What It Measures	What It Could Mean
Creatinine	Creatinine is a waste product of protein metabolism that provides insight into kidney function	• Abnormally high numbers may indicate nutritional compromise or impaired renal function
Glucose	Glucose blood levels provide insight into insulin production, nutritional status	• Hypoglycemia sometimes occurs with nutritional compromise • Hyperglycemia can indicate diabetes or renal compromise
Iron	Helps with oxygen transport within the hemoglobin	• Low iron levels in children can impair appetite, result in fatigue, and cause cravings for unusual non-food items
Sodium	Sodium is important to neuromuscular functioning and determines fluid levels in the body	• Abnormally high sodium levels can indicate dehydration • Abnormally low levels can occur with severe undernutrition
Potassium	Assists with maintenance of homeostasis and facilitates neuromuscular functioning	• Abnormally high results can indicate dehydration, renal dysfunction, or respiratory issues • Low results can indicate nutritional compromise
Albumin	Albumin is a protein in our plasma that maintains osmotic pressure in blood vessels and transports nutrients and hormones	• Abnormally low results can indicate nutritional compromise but are also present during any acute inflammatory process • Albumin often increases when clients are dehydrated
Pre-albumin/ transthyretin	Transthyretin (formerly called pre-albumin) is a protein produced by the liver that is responsible for hormone transport and is used by the body to build other proteins	• Abnormally low levels can indicate nutritional risk, zinc deficiency, GI dysfunction, or inflammation/infection

Clinical Observations

State and Sensory Regulation

You can learn a great deal by simply watching the infant or child. Do their fine motor and gross motor skills appear age appropriate? How is the child positioned? How is the child communicating? Of course, one of the first things to pay attention to is the child's state. How are they responding to sensory information in the environment? Are they becoming irritable or agitated? Are they shutting down and becoming lethargic? It is also important to note how the baby or child responds to your attempts to change that state. Can you successfully alert that lethargic, drowsy child? Are there strategies that work to calm the child who is upset and irritable (e.g., Case-Smith et al., 2015)?

Continuum of States

- **Deep sleep:** Relaxed, little to no movement, no eye movement under closed lids, may startle or jerk occasionally
- **Drowsy/light sleep:** Eye movements visible under closed lids or glassy eyes if open, mouthing movements, may exhibit vocalizations or whimpers
- **Quiet alert:** Awake and reacting to environment, minimal motor activity
- **Active alert:** Awake and reacting to environment, increased motor activity
- **Agitated:** Awake and fussing
- **Extremely dysregulated:** Intense crying, not responsive to calming attempts

Strategies for Sensory Regulation

Infants:

- Weighted blankets
- Swaddling
- Rocking
- Suckling or sucking

Children:

- Music
- Suckling, sucking, or oral play
- Deep pressure, joint compression
- Movement (e.g., swinging, jumping, rocking)
- Slow, easy breathing
- Sensory brushing

Respiration

Our first clinical impressions also include observations about respiration. Does the client appear to be working hard to breathe? What is the respiratory rate at rest? Does it appear to be within the range of normal? Does it change with activity? With speaking? With crying? To answer those questions, it is helpful to know what a normal respiratory rate looks like.

Norms for Resting Respiratory Rate in Breaths per Minute (bpm)

Typical, full-term infant: 30–49 bpm

Premature infant: 40–60 bpm (ill infant: 65+ bpm)

Children: 20–30 bpm

Adults: 15–16 bpm

Older adults: 20 bpm

In addition to watching, listen to the breathing. Do you hear wheezing? Stridor (audible breathing)? Wetness or congestion? Any of these could be indicators of underlying airway impairments (Weir et al., 2007, 2009). Is this child working hard to breathe? Look for the following signs of dyspnea at rest, when the child is crying or speaking, and during your food and utensil trials:

- Increased respiratory rate
- Inhalations mid-word or phrase; decreased number of syllables per breath
- Low vocal intensity; weak cry
- Activation of neck, upper rib cage muscles
- Holding bolus in oral cavity to take extra breaths
- Pausing between swallows to breathe

Positioning

Observations about the child's positioning can also provide us with insight into respiration. Remember that the respiratory muscles are part and parcel of the muscle set that makes up our core. A child who is demonstrating trunk weakness or instability is likely also demonstrating weakness in the respiratory musculature with subsequent inefficiencies in respiration. To determine if the child is well-positioned, ask yourself these questions:

- Are their trunk, head, and neck generally in line? Can the child maintain this alignment throughout the meal?
- Can the child move side to side and rotate at midline? What happens to respiration when they perform these movements?
- Can the child participate in feeding (e.g., reach, bring food or utensils to their mouth, hold utensils)?
- Is the respiratory rate steady? Is breath support sufficient?
- Do their lower extremities support their upper body?
- Is there support for their feet?
- Is the feeder comfortable and positioned in a way to facilitate eye contact and communication with the child?

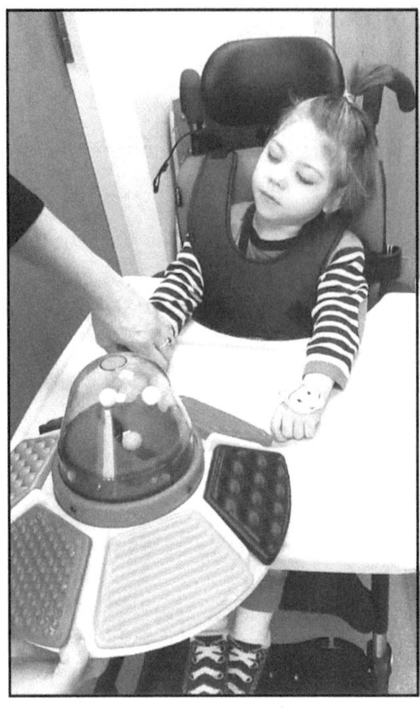

Gastrointestinal Function

A full assessment of GI function is not within the scope of practice of feeding and swallowing therapists, as this determination lies in the hands of physicians. It is true, however, that many infants and children with underlying GI issues are referred for feeding and swallowing evaluations and treatment. Why do these children end up with us? It's because GI disorders are the most common source of food refusal and feeding difficulties in infants and children (Schwarz et al., 2001; Williams et al., 2010). Clearly, as feeding specialists, we are not physicians equipped to make medical diagnoses. But as rehabilitation professionals, it is incumbent upon us to be able to recognize the signs and symptoms of GI dysfunction so we can facilitate appropriate medical referrals. What are those signs and symptoms?

Esophageal

- Chest pain or pressure
- Heartburn (more common in adolescents than infants and children)
- Regurgitation (or excessive regurgitation in infants)
- Nausea
- Water brash (i.e., excessive salivation)

Pulmonary

- Asthma (not well controlled by medication alone)
- Chronic cough
- Pneumonia
- Bronchiectasis
- Respiratory difficulties (e.g., shortness of breath, increased work of breathing)

Ear, Nose, and Throat

- Laryngitis
- Ear infections
- Sinusitis
- Throat ulcers
- Hoarseness or throat clearing
- Laryngospasm
- Paradoxical vocal fold movement

Feeding and Swallowing

- Complaints of food sticking in the throat or chest area
- Weight loss or inadequate weight gain
- Food refusal or limitations in food repertoire
- Loss of previously preferred foods from repertoire
- Gagging or choking
- Burping or belching
- Painful swallowing
- Apnea during feeding (more common in infancy)
- Arching or turning away from nipple
- Stridor or wheezing

Other

- Dental erosions or dental hypersensitivity
- Sleep disturbance
- Sleep bruxism
- Breakdown of oral mucosa (e.g., canker sores, ulcerations)
- Halitosis or acidic smell on breath

- Infrequent stooling
- Pain and effort with stooling
- Persistent irritability (particularly that which begins during feeding)

Some of our clients will undergo an instrumental assessment at the direction of their physician. An instrumental assessment of GI functioning differs from an imaging test of oral or pharyngeal swallow functioning in a significant way: There is no "gold standard" for a GI assessment. No single test exists that assesses for all possible causes of GI dysfunction. Instead, each test provides insight into one aspect of GI functioning that may nevertheless be helpful to us in treatment planning. The following table provides a description of some of these tests.

Procedure	Description	Purpose
Upper GI/barium swallow	Involves a fluoroscopy (i.e., a live, moving X-ray); Time limited given radiation exposure	Identifies anatomical abnormalities, including herniation, stricture, and malrotation
pH probe	Measures pH in the esophagus every 2–4 seconds via a 24-hour study	Provides information regarding the number and duration of *acidic* reflux episodes
Impedance testing	Measures movement within the esophagus; Sometimes combined with a pH probe	Assists with identification of *non-acidic* reflux episodes
Scintigraphy	Nuclear medicine procedure that measures gastric emptying time	Identifies delayed gastric motility
Endoscopy	Provides a visual inspection of the esophagus via endoscope	Identifies mucosal injury and allows for biopsy
Manometry	Measures timing and strength of esophageal muscle contractions via a catheter placed trans-nasally into the esophagus	Provides information regarding esophageal peristalsis and upper and lower esophageal sphincter functioning; Assists in the identification of spasm and achalasia

Oral and Pharyngeal Swallow Function

An assessment of oral and pharyngeal swallow function is typically accomplished in two parts: clinical assessment and, if needed, instrumental assessment. A *clinical assessment* provides us with information regarding oral motor function, utensil use, self-feeding skills, and responses to a variety of food and liquid types. Importantly, it also identifies the signs and symptoms of aspiration and pharyngeal dysphagia. In contrast, an *instrumental assessment* allows for the visualization of the pharyngeal anatomy and physiology so we can identify specific physiological impairments.

Clinical Assessment

1. **Oral Mechanism Examination**

   Our clinical assessment typically begins with a look at the mouth. Ideally, we would like the child to imitate a variety of jaw, lip, and tongue movements for us, but if that's not possible given the child's age, cognitive ability, or attention, then we have to make judgments about oral functioning at rest and during feeding and speech activities. Here's what to pay attention to:

   a. **Jaw:** Can the child...

      - Open and close their mouth fully?
      - Open and close their mouth quickly?
      - Open and close their mouth against resistance you provide?
      - Grade their jaw movements (i.e., vary their mouth opening depending on the size and shape of the bolus or in response to verbal command)?
      - Open their mouth without moving their tongue?

   Watch for weakness, instability, or impairment in function:

      - Signs of pain or discomfort with movement
      - Limitations in range of motion
      - Associated head movements as the jaw moves
      - Jaw shifting during graded movements
      - Jaw retraction or thrust
      - Bite reflex

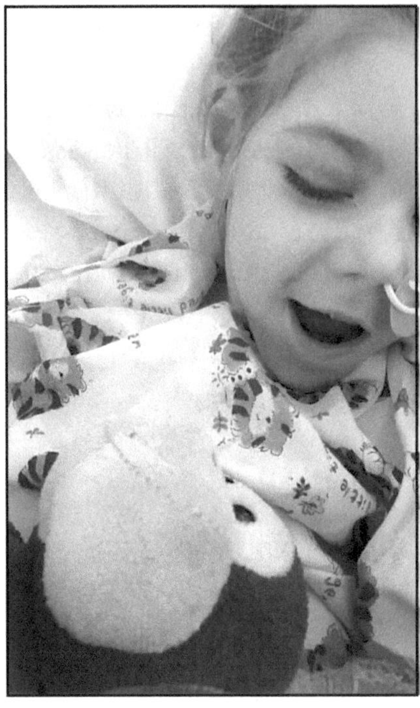

b. **Tongue:** Can the child…

- Move their tongue to their top lip, bottom lip, and the corners of their mouth?
- Move their tongue across midline intraorally?
- Lick their lips completely?
- Touch their tongue to the alveolar ridge?
- Protrude their tongue past their lips?
- Move their tongue without associated jaw or lip movements?

Watch for weakness or impairment in function:

- Limitations in range of motion or function
- Associated head or jaw movements when moving their tongue
- Midline stop during lateralization
- Tongue thrust
- Tongue retraction
- Limited protrusion or tongue tie

c. **Lips:** Can the child…

- Retract their lips fully?
- Close their lips tightly?
- Purse their lips?
- Move their lips without associated tongue movements?

Watch for weakness or impairment in function:

- Inability to move through the full range of motion
- Inability to move lips without associated tongue movements
- Consistent lip retraction

d. **Oral health assessment:**

- What is the condition of the mucosa (e.g., dry/cracked or pink/moist)?
- Is the child experiencing any oral pain or discomfort?
- What is the condition of their lips and tongue (e.g., moist, dry, coated?)
- Do their teeth appear clean? Is there discoloration? Do you see obvious dental decay?
- Does saliva production appear adequate? Excessive?
- What child or maternal risk factors for poor oral health are present?*

Maternal Risk Factors	Child Risk Factors
• Mother or primary caregiver had active decay in the past 12 months • Mother or primary caregiver does not have a dentist	• Continual bottle or sippy cup use with fluid other than water • Frequent snacking • Special health care needs • White spots or visible decalcifications in the past 12 months • Obvious decay • Visible plaque accumulation • Gingivitis (swollen/bleeding gums)

* The American Academy of Pediatrics has developed an oral health assessment tool for pediatric practitioners that is available at https://www.aap.org/en-us/Documents/oralhealth_RiskAssessmentTool.pdf

2. Cranial Nerve Assessment

A cranial nerve assessment is an easy way to obtain information about your client's neurological functioning. An examination of the cranial nerves listed here can assist you in identifying neurological deficits that directly impact oral and sensory functions of feeding and swallowing.

Cranial Nerve	Function	Assessment in Infants	Assessment in Children
Trigeminal (V)	• Motor (jaw movement for chewing and biting) • Sensory (upper face, upper lip)	• Touch child's face and observe for rooting • Touch child's gums and observe for phasic bite • Look for tonic bite • Look for impaired jaw movements	• Observe child when opening and closing mouth and when biting • Palpate masseter muscles bilaterally during bite • Look for impaired jaw movements
Facial nerve (VII)	• Motor (jaw movement, facial muscles) • Sensory (taste perception in the front and middle tongue)	• Touch front tongue and lips, and observe for tongue protrusion • Look for asymmetry in facial movements and absent rooting	• Observe during lip retraction • Explore ability to identify tastes* • Look for facial asymmetry

Cranial Nerve	Function	Assessment in Infants	Assessment in Children
Glossopharyngeal (IX) and vagus (X) (assessed together)	• Motor (pharyngeal muscles for gagging and swallowing; laryngeal function) • Sensory (pharynx; taste perception in the posterior tongue and tongue base)	• Observe for gag** and swallow response • Listen for hoarse cry • Look for palatal weakness	• Observe for gag** and swallow response • Listen for hoarse voice • Look for palatal weakness
Accessory (XI)	• Motor (neck muscles)	• Touch child's face and observe head turn during rooting response	• Observe head turning side to side; shrug shoulders and look for weakness, slowness
Hypoglossal (XII)	• Motor (tongue movements)	• Insert gloved finger in mouth and observe for suckle response	• Observe during tongue protrusion • Listen for imprecise articulation

* Taste is not always an accurate tool for assessing cranial nerve function in children. First, there is considerable overlap in cranial nerve function for taste perception. Second, children with sensory processing difficulties often have altered taste perception, which limits their ability to accurately identify tastes.

** Caution is advised in the assessment of the gag response in children. We are often working with children who have had unpleasurable experiences (to say the least) with food and oral input. It is important to be sensitive to that, especially upon first meeting the child. **Never force your way into a child's mouth.**

3. Considerations for Infants

a. Infant reflexes are critical building blocks for successful feeding. As always, it is important to proceed slowly and to wait for the baby to invite you into their mouth. Look for the following:

- **Rooting reflex:** Assess by touching their lower lip or cheek. Watch for the baby's mouth to open in response and for their head to turn toward the touch.
- **Sucking reflex:** Assess by placing your (gloved) finger on the baby's tongue. Feel for the tongue cupping around your finger. Is the suckle rhythmic? Is the suction strong?
- **Phasic bite:** Assess by touching the lateral gums. Watch for a firm bite. A strong bite that is difficult for the baby to release is more tonic in nature and considered abnormal.
- **Transverse tongue reflex:** Assess by touching the sides of their tongue. Watch for lateral tongue movement.

b. Look for tethered oral tissue during your examination of the infant's oral cavity. Be sure to do a visual check for tongue- and lip-ties, as well as a *functional* assessment (Mills & Ashford, 2008; Mills et al., 2019; O'Shea et al., 2017). In other words, even if the tongue appears tethered, what is the impact on function? Can the baby cup their tongue when crying? Does the tongue tip reach the alveolar ridge? Can the baby protrude their tongue between their lips? Did you notice any restriction in movement during your assessment of the suck response? Does the mother report difficulties with latch or pain with breastfeeding? Do you see reduced upper lip flanging during feeding?

c. You can assess for non-nutritive sucking by having the baby suck on your gloved finger or observing the baby with a pacifier. Non-nutritive sucking ability does not predict nutritive sucking potential but does give us some insight into the infant's neurological maturation. Infants use non-nutritive sucking for a variety of purposes, most importantly for calming. We know that non-nutritive sucking reduces stress and improves behavioral state. It facilitates gastric motility by increasing saliva swallows and can help reduce apnea.

Interpreting Oral Assessment Results

Observation	Implication
Face: Asymmetry of lips, face, tongue, palate	Likely underlying neurological impairment
Face/oral cavity: Open-mouth resting posture	Possible nasal airway obstruction or possible hypotonia
Oral cavity: White color at junction of soft and hard palate	Possible submucosal cleft
Oral cavity: Red mucosa	Inflammation, irritation
Oral cavity: Translucent palate	Possible submucosal cleft
Oral cavity: High, vaulted palate	Possible impaired lingual-palatal contact (may be the result of intubation in infancy)
Oral cavity: Excessive saliva, drooling	Possible swallow impairment, low tone, or impaired lip closure; May also be related to reflux (water brash)
Oral cavity: Dry mucosa	Possible dehydration or medication side effects
Teeth: Discolored teeth, visible plaque	Poor oral hygiene and dental health
Jaw: Jaw shifting during graded movements	Jaw instability
Jaw: Jaw retraction or thrust	Underlying instability (check stability of head, neck, and trunk)
Jaw: Bite reflex	Underlying instability (check stability of head, neck, and trunk)
Lips/tongue: Associated jaw or head movement when moving lips or tongue	Incomplete differentiation (check for jaw instability)
Tongue: Limited tongue protrusion	Possible tongue tie or hypertonia
Tongue: Inability to move tongue across midline without midline stop	Underlying jaw instability
Tongue: Tongue deviation	Likely underlying neurological impairment
Lips: Lip retraction at rest	Underlying instability (check stability of jaw, head, and neck)
Infant reflexes: Absent root, suckle, or phasic bite in infant	Underlying neurological impairment (may be related to prematurity)
Voice: Hoarse voice, cry	Possible cranial nerve impairment (IX, X) or vocal fold paralysis (check for history of neurological impairment or laryngeal trauma)

4. Food and Utensil Trials

This is our opportunity to observe the child with a variety of utensils, foods, and liquids to see what's working and not working. Regardless of which food or utensil you choose to begin with, our framework is going to be the same: Does or can the child accept the bolus or utensil? Is the child interested? Aware of the task demands? What happens in the child's mouth? Can the child manage the demands of this particular bolus type or utensil? Does the swallow appear safe and timely? Are there clinical signs of aspiration? What happened after the swallow? Was there residue in the mouth? Is the child aware of it? Doing something about it?

a. **Suckle and suck:** Whether the baby is bottle-fed or breastfed, we want to assess latch and initiation of suckle and suck. Is the baby exhibiting good suck-swallow-breathe coordination? Or are you seeing stress behaviors suggestive of respiratory fatigue or air hunger? Watch for fluctuations in performance over the course of the feeding. Does the baby fatigue? Become less coordinated as the feeding progresses?

Stress Behaviors

- Changes in state (e.g., lethargy or fussiness)
- Autonomic changes (e.g., changes in respiratory rate, heart rate, oxygen saturation)
- Motor restlessness, limb tension, splayed fingers
- Fatigue, slowing
- Grimacing, nasal flaring, chin tugging
- Hiccups
- Stridor, gurgling
- Limited intake
- Coughing, choking, gulping
- Wet, congested respiration

b. **Puree via spoon:** We want to evaluate the child using whatever spoon they typically use at home. If this is an initial attempt at spoon feeding, choose a spoon that has a fairly shallow bowl to make clearance as easy as possible to start. As you observe spoon feeding, ask yourself:

- Does the child open their mouth in anticipation of the spoon or food?
- Does the child open their mouth with sufficient opening to accept the spoon? Is their mouth opening too wide for the spoon? Not wide enough? In other words, are you seeing evidence of graded jaw movements?
- Does the child clear the spoon with their lips? With their teeth? Or is the feeder actually clearing the spoon for the child by using upward movement? Does the spoon bowl seem too deep for this child?
- Does the child use their tongue to move the food backward for swallow? Or is there forward tongue protrusion? If so, do these movements actually push the food out of the mouth?
- Does the swallow occur? Are there any signs of aspiration?
- Is there any residue? Is the child aware of it? Do they make any effort to clear it?
- Does respiratory rate or work of breathing increase?

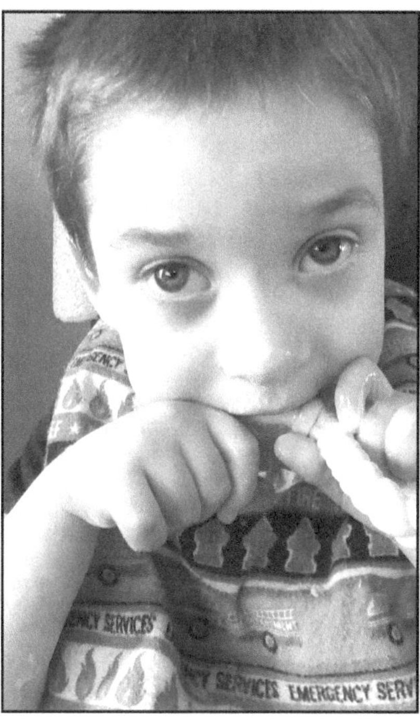

c. **Liquids via cup:** As with spoon feeding, we want to observe the child using whatever cup (or cups) they typically use. If this is going to be the child's first attempt at cup drinking, choose a cup that will allow you to slow the flow, such as a covered cup or a small open cup that you can control. As you observe cup drinking, ask yourself:

- Does the child open their mouth in anticipation of the cup? Is their mouth opening sufficient? Too wide? Not wide enough?
- Does the child use their lips to close on the cup? Or is the child biting on the cup to maintain stability?
- Does the child manage the liquid flow with efficient tongue movements? Is there liquid loss? When does it occur?
- Does the swallow occur? Are there any signs of aspiration?
- Is there any residue? Is the child aware of it? Do they make any effort to clear it?
- Does respiratory rate or work of breathing increase?
- Are there differences with different liquid viscosities?

d. **Liquids via straw:** To start, use a straw that has a typical diameter and length. If the child is having difficulty drawing liquid through the straw, you can shorten it or use a straw with a one-way valve. (See chapter 5 for more details.) As you observe straw drinking, ask yourself:

- Does the child close their lips completely around the straw?
- Does the child draw liquid through the length of the straw successfully?
- Does the child keep their tongue retracted during straw drinking? Or do you see the tongue coming forward to suckle the straw?
- Does the child take serial swallows via the straw? Or only single sips?
- Does the swallow occur? Are there any signs of aspiration?
- Is there any residue? Is the child aware of it? Do they make any effort to clear it?

- Does work of breathing or respiratory rate increase? Does this occur with serial swallowing only or with single sips as well?
- Are there differences with different liquid viscosities?

e. **Chewables/biteables:** As always, start with foods the child is eating at home or school. As you think about trials of novel foods, let your assessment of the child's oral motor function guide your choices. If you observed little to no tongue lateralization or limited jaw opening and closing, then this is a child who is unlikely to be able to manage chewable foods. Instead, trials of more easily dissolvable solids (e.g., freeze-dried fruit, puffs) would be more appropriate for assessment. As you observe biting and chewing, ask yourself:

- Does the child readily accept the food from you or self-feed independently?
- Does the child open their mouth in anticipation of the food?
- Does the child use their tongue to move the food laterally onto the teeth? Do they move food from right to left and left to right with their tongue? Is there a midline stop as they do so?
- Does the child use rotary movements for chewing? Or do you see largely vertical jaw movement? Are these movements efficient or not?
- Does the child keep their lips closed during chewing?
- Does the swallow occur? Are there any signs of choking or aspiration?
- Is there any residue? Is the child aware of it? Do they make any effort to clear it? How successful are those efforts?
- Does work of breathing or respiratory rate increase? Does this vary with the amount of chewing required?

Clinical Signs and Symptoms of Aspiration

Infants:

- Wheezing, stridor
- Bluish color around lips
- Recurrent pneumonia, bronchitis, or respiratory difficulties
- Apnea
- Changes in heart rate
- Increased respiratory rate or effort
- Grimacing or nasal flaring
- Increased respiratory mucus or respiratory congestion
- Wet vocal quality
- Wet, congested respiration
- Changes in state (e.g., lethargy, irritability)
- Fatigue, slowing
- Nipple refusal
- Coughing, choking, sputtering, or gulping

Children:

- Wheezing, stridor
- Coughing, choking
- Recurrent pneumonia, bronchitis, or respiratory difficulties
- Increased respiratory rate or effort
- Increased respiratory mucus or respiratory congestion
- Wet vocal quality
- Wet, congested respiration
- Changes in state (e.g., lethargy, irritability)
- Fatigue, slowing
- Hoarseness
- Limited intake

5. Child-Caregiver Interactions

We can gather a lot of information about the nature of our client's feeding difficulties by watching the child with their parents or caregivers during mealtimes. For those of us working in schools or clinics, it can be difficult to simulate a natural feeding environment, but observing the parents and the child together can provide us with information about how the child typically performs. In addition to parents, feeders may be grandparents, aides and assistants, teachers, daycare providers, babysitters, friends, or any number of other people close to the child. Assess as many of these interactions as possible to obtain information about performance fluctuations, identify any impacts on performance, and round out your overall impression of the child.

As you watch the parents feed the child or interact with the child while they eat, observe the following:

a. **Communication:** Do the feeder and the child demonstrate effective eye contact and communication? Does the child signal their hunger? How do they do that? Does the feeder recognize those signals and respond? What is the nature of the verbal communication? Does the feeder have to coax and negotiate with the child? Does the feeder have to use distractions (like screens) to increase intake? Does the feeder comment positively where appropriate? Does the child communicate nonverbally (e.g., with facial expressions, gestures)? If so, is the feeder able to interpret that communication? Is the pace appropriate? If not, is the child able to communicate that to the feeder? How does the child signal that they are full? Does the feeder interpret that signal appropriately?

b. **Food choices:** Are the food types being offered age appropriate? Are they appropriate to the child's feeding skill? Are bite sizes appropriate? What utensils does the feeder offer? Are they appropriate to the child's age and feeding skill? Which foods are accepted by the child? What happens if the child refuses? How does the feeder respond? Is the child encouraged to self-feed?

c. **Positioning:** How is the child positioned? Do they appear comfortable? If not, is the feeder able to make appropriate adjustments?

d. **Modeling and cueing:** Does the feeder model appropriate eating behaviors and provide cues to the child when needed? How does the child respond to those cues?

Instrumental Assessment

Clinical assessment can certainly alert us to the various signs and symptoms of aspiration, but it cannot definitively tell us what is happening in the pharynx. In order to fully assess pharyngeal function and airway protection, we need to view the pharynx and airway during actual swallowing—and that means we need an instrumental assessment.

Your client needs an instrumental assessment of swallow function when:

- You have identified signs and symptoms of aspiration during your clinical assessment.
- You are concerned about silent aspiration.
- You need guidance regarding diet options, utensils, or strategies.
- You need information about pharyngeal physiology to guide your treatment plan.

Instrumental assessment for babies and children typically takes two forms: *modified barium swallow* (MBS) studies, which are most common, or *flexible (fiberoptic) endoscopic evaluation of swallow* (FEES) studies. Regardless of the type of test that is available or is chosen, it is important to understand the purposes and limitations of instrumental assessment.

Instrumental Assessment

Instrumental assessment can:

- Allow us to view and assess the anatomy and physiology of the pharynx (and depending on the test, the esophagus)
- Help us identify the physiological cause of the dysphagia
- Detect laryngeal penetration and aspiration
- Assess differences between bolus and utensil types
- Assess the efficacy of compensatory strategies (e.g., slowing the flow rate, reducing the bolus size, pacing)

Instrumental assessment does not:

- Rule out aspiration (It can only tell us that our client did not aspirate this day, under these conditions.)
- Determine the impact of the dysphagia on the child or predict which child will develop pneumonia or other health consequences as a result of their dysphagia
- Simulate mealtimes (This is *not* real-life eating!)

Let's break it down by study. An MBS study is done via videofluoroscopy, which is a live, moving X-ray that allow us to visualize food and liquid as it moves from the oral cavity, through the pharynx, and into the esophagus. MBS studies are generally completed in hospital radiology departments, although they are occasionally accomplished via mobile units in some areas of the country. The client is positioned in the fluoroscope and consumes food and liquid that has been mixed with barium. The barium allows for visualization of the boluses under X-ray. Because of the radiation exposure involved, the test is very time sensitive and generally only allows for one or two trials of each food or liquid.

Modified Barium Swallow (MBS) Test

Questions this test answers:

- Did aspiration occur? Why did it occur?
- Did my client respond to the aspiration? If so, how? Cough? Throat clear? Change in respiration? Change in vocal quality? Something else?
- Which strategies or maneuvers were attempted? Which ones were effective?
- What utensils were tried? Were there differences in swallow function with different utensils?
- What is the recommended diet level (and why)?

Questions this test does *not* answer:

- What is the condition of the pharynx or larynx? (X-ray does not allow us to examine the soft tissue or cartilage effectively.)
- What will happen under conditions different from the test situation (e.g., when the child is positioned differently, more distracted, or more fatigued)?
- What changes happen over the course of a meal?
- What are the effects of fatigue or low endurance?

In contrast, an FEES test is completed via endoscope. A flexible, fiberoptic endoscope is passed through the client's nose and into the pharynx, giving the clinician a "birds-eye" view of the pharynx and airway during swallowing. There is a brief period of "white out" or image loss at the height of the swallow as the movement within the pharynx reflects the light from the endoscope. Food and liquid swallows are completed with the endoscope in place. Only the pharyngeal phase of the swallow is visible. FEES units are portable, so the test not have to take place within the hospital. There is no radiation exposure, but clinicians are sensitive to the potential discomfort associated with the endoscope, which can limit the number of trials completed.

Fiberoptic Endoscopic Evaluation of Swallowing (FEES) Test

Questions this test answers:

- Did aspiration occur? If so, why?
- What was the client's response to the aspiration?
- What does the larynx look like? Is it functioning to protect the airway?
- Were there any mucosal changes in the pharynx or larynx? Redness? Swelling? Irritation?
- What strategies or maneuvers were attempted? Which ones were effective?
- What utensils were tried? Were there differences in swallow function with different utensils?
- What is the recommended diet level (and why?)

Questions this test does *not* answer:

- Were there issues with oral transit? Mastication? Oral bolus management?
- Were there issues with esophageal clearance? Reflux?
- What happens over the course of an entire mealtime?

	Advantages	Limitations
Modified barium swallow study	• Best test to assess transition from oral cavity, through pharynx, and into esophagus • Good view of hyolaryngeal excursion	• Time limited due to radiation exposure • Positioning constraints • Child must accept/ consume barium • Limited ability to assess for mucosal irritation and breakdown • Limited view of vocal fold function
Flexible (fiberoptic) endoscopic evaluation of swallow	• Able to use real foods • No positioning constraints • Best test to assess airway and vocal fold function • Allows for assessment during breastfeeding • Allows for assessment of aspiration of saliva	• Unable to assess oral bolus management or esophageal clearance • Client must tolerate endoscope • Brief image loss at height of swallow

An instrumental assessment is not meant to stand alone. It is meant to be integrated into all of the other clinical observations and assessments we have completed. However, that isn't always easy to do. Instrumental and clinical assessments are often done by different clinicians, in different places, on different days. **Therefore, it is crucial for the primary therapist (who is making the referral) and the evaluating therapist (who is completing the instrumental assessment) to communicate with each other in order to effectively integrate the assessment results.** The referring clinician has the responsibility to communicate to the evaluating therapist information about the signs and symptoms of aspiration that have been observed. Why is this child being referred for a swallow study? What are the observations from the clinical assessment? The referring team can also provide information about positioning concerns, current diet, and preferred utensils.

The clinician performing the swallow study has the responsibility to visualize and describe pharyngeal anatomy and physiology in light of the clinical concerns. It is also the responsibility of the evaluating therapist to link the observations about physiology with those clinical concerns. Let's say the child's early intervention team has communicated concerns about coughing with eating and drinking. The evaluating clinician completes the swallow study and notes delays in swallow response and slowed laryngeal closure. But how does that change in physiology connect to the clinical observations? Was that cough noted during the assessment? Was it associated with aspiration? What was the clinical response to the aspiration, if it did indeed occur?

The following pages contain examples of communication forms to facilitate collaboration between the primary and evaluating clinicians when referring a client for a swallow study.

Clinician Form

Modified Barium Swallow Study Referral Form

Client name: ______________________ Date of birth: ____________

Date of referral: __________ Date of study (if known): __________

Parent/caregiver contact information: ______________________________

____

Medical diagnosis: ____

____

Pertinent medical history: ______________________________________

____

Positioning concerns: ____

____

Current diet: ____

____

Current utensil use: ____

____

Clinical signs/symptoms observed: _______________________________

____

Specific questions/concerns for the study: _________________________

____

Referring clinician: ____

Phone: ______________________ Email: _____________________

Clinician Form

Modified Barium Swallow Study Results Form

Client name: ____________________ Date of birth: _____________

Date of study: ____________

____________________ participated in a modified barium swallow study today. Below are the preliminary results.

Food/liquid and utensils trialed: ______________________________

____

Description of Swallow Physiology

Oral phase:

- ☐ Impaired suck/suckle
- ☐ Impaired velopharyngeal closure
- ☐ Impaired lingual propulsion
- ☐ Impaired mastication
- ☐ Impaired oral containment
- ☐ Other _____________

Pharyngeal phase:

- ☐ Delayed swallow response
- ☐ Impaired hyolaryngeal excursion
- ☐ Residue in _________________
- ☐ Aspiration of ______________
- ☐ Impaired laryngeal closure
- ☐ Impaired tongue base retraction
- ☐ Impaired pharyngeal motility

Clinical response to aspiration:

- ☐ None (silent)
- ☐ Cough without airway clearance
- ☐ Change in respiration
- ☐ Cough with airway clearance
- ☐ Throat clearing
- ☐ Other _____________

Diet Recommendations

☐ Food ________________ ☐ Liquid ________________

Utensil Recommendations

☐ Bottle _________ ☐ Cup ________ ☐ Other _________

Feeding Recommendations

☐ Slow pace/external pacing

☐ Bite/sip size ___________

☐ Other ________________

Please feel free to contact me with any questions you have.

Clinician: ________________

Phone: __________________ Email: _____________________

Parent/Caregiver Handout

Modified Barium Swallow Study: What Do I Need to Know?

1. **What is it?**

   A modified barium swallow (MBS) study—also known as a swallow function test, a video swallow study, or a videofluoroscopic swallow study—is a test done in radiology using videofluoroscopy, which is a live, moving X-ray. It allows us to see the swallow muscles at work during actual swallowing. It allows us to look for aspiration (i.e., food or liquid going down "the wrong pipe") and residue (i.e., food or liquid "sticking" in the throat), but it can also give us information about *why* these problems are occurring. We can often identify weakness, slowness, discoordination, and decreased sensation.

2. **When is it appropriate?**

   These studies are helpful at different points during the treatment process. They are sometimes done before treatment starts as a way to gather information that will guide the treatment plan. They are sometimes done intermittently, such as when a change in diet is planned or if swallow function appears to have changed.

3. **How is it done?**

   The child is positioned in a chair that allows them to sit in their typical feeding position. Foods mixed with barium and liquid barium of different thicknesses are given to the child to eat or drink. Whenever possible, familiar cups, spoons, and foods are used to make the child more comfortable and to ensure we have a picture of "typical" feeding. As problems are identified, changes in bite size, positioning, texture, and so on are made to determine what will make the child as safe as possible during eating and drinking.

4. **How long does it take?**

   The test itself takes just a few minutes, but it does take some time to get the child properly positioned and ready to go. In general, families should plan to spend between 30 to 60 minutes at the hospital.

5. **Do I have to do anything to prepare?**

   The child does not have to fast prior to the study and can take any regularly scheduled medications, but we do ask that they come somewhat hungry so they are able to eat and drink during the study.

6. **What should I bring?**

   Bring the cup and spoon your child is most familiar with. The therapist may also ask you to bring along some particular foods. Bring something your child is likely to want to eat. You can also bring music, small toys, or books that will make your child more comfortable.

7. **What happens when the study is done?**

   The therapist and radiologist will review the images and put together a report. Results are generally provided on the day of the study, but the full written report likely will be completed and available in one to two days. The therapist will use the information from the study to guide further treatment decisions regarding safe foods, liquids, and utensils as well as decisions regarding appropriate treatment techniques.

Once we have completed clinical and instrumental assessment of swallow function, we aren't ready to move forward with our management plan until we have put the aspiration risk in context—that is, in the context of the child's potential for pulmonary clearance and risk of illness (Hirsch et al., 2016). To do so, we must consider a variety of factors, including the child's overall medical condition and medical stability, nutritional status (to gauge immune system function), hydration status (to gauge cilia movement), pulmonary status, and oral hygiene. (See "Aspiration and Illness" in chapter 1 for a full description of risk factors for aspiration-related illness.)

Sensory Responses

Think about a bacon cheeseburger. Yummy, right? A hamburger covered with cheese, bacon, lettuce, tomato, and maybe pickles too. On the bun, there's ketchup and mustard or maybe mayonnaise instead, depending on your preference. The bun might be toasted or doughy. Maybe it has sesame seeds on it. Does that sound delicious to you? If you're a child with a sensory processing disorder, that burger is actually a terrifying mix of sensory experiences. The taste of the hamburger, combined with the cheese and bacon, and mixed with the taste of the condiments, creates a variety of sensory demands, each one more difficult than the last.

Each bite tastes different than the one before it, depending on how much pickle or ketchup you get. Each bite also feels different than the one before it, depending on how much bun or meat you get. And the smells! Meats, cheese, and mustard, all in combination with one another. What about the textures? The meat may be hard to chew, while the pickle is mushy. And the cheese is melted, but the bun is toasted and crunchy with hard bits on top. And we haven't even factored in the other foods on the plate, the utensils, or any of the other sensory information in the environment!

That's an awful lot of information to process, isn't it? That's what we're asking ourselves to do multiple times a day, and for those of us with typically functioning sensory systems, it's easy. In fact, it's pleasurable. However, that's not the case for children with sensory processing disorders.

We generally categorize sensory processing disorders into the following subtypes:

Sensory Over-Responsive/ Hypersensitive	Sensory Under-Responsive/ Hyposensitive	Sensory Craving/Seeking
• Faster, more intense responses to sensory input • Responses last for longer periods of time • Seek escape from environmental stimuli	• Slower, less intense responses to sensory input • Little exploration of the environment	• Strong desire for sensory input • Unusual preferences

Not surprisingly, there is evidence to support a link between sensory processing disorders and feeding disorders (Nadon et al., 2011; Zobel-Lachiusa et al., 2015). Children with sensory processing disorders are more likely to exhibit food refusal, have limitations in their food repertoire, and exhibit rigidity about what, where, when, with what utensil, and with whom they eat. This rigidity makes trying new foods difficult. It makes eating in new places, like at a friend's house or a birthday party, a challenge.

Assessment of feeding in children with sensory processing disorders is best done via inventory and observation. Ask parents to provide information about what foods the child always eats, sometimes eats, and never eats. The sample food inventory on the next page can help parents track this information. A diet diary can be helpful in this regard as well.

Parent/Caregiver Worksheet

Sample Food Inventory

Please indicate the foods your child always eats, sometimes eats, and never eats, including the frequency with which different foods are eaten.

FRUITS	All the time	Most of the time	Occasionally	Rarely	Never
1. ____________	1	2	3	4	5
2. ____________	1	2	3	4	5
3. ____________	1	2	3	4	5
4. ____________	1	2	3	4	5
5. ____________	1	2	3	4	5
6. ____________	1	2	3	4	5
7. ____________	1	2	3	4	5
8. ____________	1	2	3	4	5
9. ____________	1	2	3	4	5
10. ____________	1	2	3	4	5

VEGETABLES	All the time	Most of the time	Occasionally	Rarely	Never
1. ____________	1	2	3	4	5
2. ____________	1	2	3	4	5
3. ____________	1	2	3	4	5
4. ____________	1	2	3	4	5
5. ____________	1	2	3	4	5
6. ____________	1	2	3	4	5
7. ____________	1	2	3	4	5
8. ____________	1	2	3	4	5
9. ____________	1	2	3	4	5
10. ____________	1	2	3	4	5

MEATS	All the time	Most of the time	Occasionally	Rarely	Never
1. ______________	1	2	3	4	5
2. ______________	1	2	3	4	5
3. ______________	1	2	3	4	5
4. ______________	1	2	3	4	5
5. ______________	1	2	3	4	5
6. ______________	1	2	3	4	5
7. ______________	1	2	3	4	5
8. ______________	1	2	3	4	5
9. ______________	1	2	3	4	5
10. ______________	1	2	3	4	5

STARCHES	All the time	Most of the time	Occasionally	Rarely	Never
1. ______________	1	2	3	4	5
2. ______________	1	2	3	4	5
3. ______________	1	2	3	4	5
4. ______________	1	2	3	4	5
5. ______________	1	2	3	4	5
6. ______________	1	2	3	4	5
7. ______________	1	2	3	4	5
8. ______________	1	2	3	4	5
9. ______________	1	2	3	4	5
10. ______________	1	2	3	4	5

CONDIMENTS	All the time	Most of the time	Occasionally	Rarely	Never
1. ____________	1	2	3	4	5
2. ____________	1	2	3	4	5
3. ____________	1	2	3	4	5
4. ____________	1	2	3	4	5
5. ____________	1	2	3	4	5
6. ____________	1	2	3	4	5
7. ____________	1	2	3	4	5
8. ____________	1	2	3	4	5
9. ____________	1	2	3	4	5
10. ____________	1	2	3	4	5

BEVERAGES	All the time	Most of the time	Occasionally	Rarely	Never
1. ____________	1	2	3	4	5
2. ____________	1	2	3	4	5
3. ____________	1	2	3	4	5
4. ____________	1	2	3	4	5
5. ____________	1	2	3	4	5
6. ____________	1	2	3	4	5
7. ____________	1	2	3	4	5
8. ____________	1	2	3	4	5
9. ____________	1	2	3	4	5
10. ____________	1	2	3	4	5

To determine sensory preferences, it can also be helpful to observe the child with familiar and novel or non-preferred foods and utensils. How does the child respond to the foods and utensils? Which are upsetting or not well tolerated? Which are preferred, well accepted, or sought out? Are there certain types of input that are particularly calming or irritating? As we complete these observations, it's important to consider tactile input, texture, taste, and smells. We are looking for patterns of response, both during our observations and as we review the inventories. Does the child prefer crunchy foods? Soft foods only? Highly flavored foods? Neutral temperatures only?

Sensory input is received not only from the external environment but internally as well. In particular, interoception is the way we process internal sensations. *Interoception* is a neurologically regulated process that allows us to recognize when we need to urinate or move our bowels, when we are cold and need to put on a sweater, when we are in pain, and—most importantly from a feeding perspective—when we are hungry or thirsty (Ceunen et al., 2016; Craig, 2002).

Children with sensory processing disorders often have difficulty with these internal sensations, so the phrase "She'll eat when she's hungry" doesn't apply if the child doesn't know she's hungry. Therefore, in addition to observing our clients while they eat and interact with foods, we want to be on the lookout for evidence of impairments in interoception. Does the mother report that her child "never gets cold" and won't wear a coat? Does the father describe the child as a "tough cookie" who hardly ever reacts when he gets hurt? Has toilet training been a struggle? It's possible, then, that hunger and satiation signals are not being processed very efficiently either.

Environment(al) Matters

Feeding and swallowing therapists work in a variety of environments, and those environments have implications for the assessment process. Early intervention therapists work in clients' homes, which affords them the opportunity for real-life functional assessment. The focus is on the family's priorities and preferences, which may or may not be related to aspiration or other swallow safety issues. In contrast, therapists who work in medical settings have opportunities for instrumental assessment and collaboration with other medical professionals. However, swallow safety is often the priority in medical settings, which can make it difficult to create a naturalistic feeding environment.

For those therapists working in school settings, where there is clearly an educational focus, it can also be more challenging to conduct a feeding and swallowing assessment. The school team is not always adequately prepared to assess and manage medically complex children with aspiration risk or significantly restricted food repertoires. But children spend a great deal of time in school. Mealtimes and snack times are a regular part of the school day and provide opportunities for the assessment and treatment of feeding and swallowing impairments. School staff certainly have an obligation to keep students safe during eating, and students must be adequately nourished in order to attend school regularly and access the curriculum.

The form on the next page can help you conduct a thorough evaluation of a child's feeding and swallowing behaviors across a variety of different settings. When conducting the assessment, though, keep in mind the setting in which you are working and how that might impact your observations.

Clinician Form

Feeding and Swallowing Evaluation Checklist

Client name: ______________________ DOB/age: _____________

General Observations

Behavior: ☐ Cooperative ☐ Resistant ☐ Refusing

Alertness: ☐ Alert ☐ Lethargic ☐ Irritable

Observations regarding self-regulation/self-calming: ___________

____

Follows directions: ☐ Verbal ☐ Gestural ☐ Not able

Vision concerns: ____

____

Hearing concerns: ____

____

Parent-child interactions: __________________________________

____

Positioning

How and where positioned: __________________________________

____

Concerns regarding: ☐ Trunk ☐ Head ☐ Extremity movement

Breathing

At rest: ☐ Normal ☐ Mouth breathing ☐ Audible/labored
☐ Congestion ☐ Stridor

With eating: ☐ Normal ☐ Mouth breathing ☐ Audible/labored
☐ Congestion ☐ Stridor

Comments: ____

____

Vocal Quality

Sound: ☐ Wet prior to eating ☐ Hoarse ☐ Breathy
☐ Weak ☐ Monopitch

Changes with eating: ______________________________

____

Drooling

Amount and frequency: ______________________________

____

Client awareness regarding drooling: ______________________________

____

Oral Mechanism

Reflexes noted: ☐ Gag ☐ Bite ☐ Rooting ☐ Swallow

Comments: ______________________________

____

Sensory Responses

Body: ______________________________

____

Face: ______________________________

____

Lips: ______________________________

____

Intraoral: ______________________________

____

Oral Movements

Jaw: ☐ Strength ☐ Mobility ☐ Bite
☐ Differentiated from lip ☐ Differentiated from tongue

Comments: ______________________________

____

Tongue: ☐ Elevation ☐ Lateralization (intraoral) ☐ Protrusion
☐ Differentiation from jaw ☐ Differentiation from lips

Comments: ____

____

Lips: ☐ Rounding ☐ Retraction ☐ Differentiation

Comments: ____

____

Teeth: ☐ Decay/discoloration ☐ Missing teeth
☐ Adequate occlusion

Comments: ____

____

Palate: ☐ Fistula/cleft ☐ Arch height/width ______________
☐ Color/appearance ______________________________

Comments: ____

____

Food Trials

Liquids: ☐ Thin ☐ Slightly thin ☐ Mildly thick
☐ Moderately thick ☐ Extremely thick

Via: ☐ Cup/type ____________ ☐ Bottle/type ____________

Observations: ☐ Suckle ☐ Suck ☐ Tongue-forward posture
☐ Tongue thrust
☐ Mouth opening ____________________________
☐ Stabilizes cup with _________________________
☐ Mouth/lip closure around cup
☐ Liquid loss _______________________________
☐ Coordination of breathing, swallowing _________
☐ Signs/symptoms of aspiration ________________

Comments: ____

____

Spoon Feeding

Food(s): ____

____

Spoon type: ____

____

Observations:
- ☐ Aware of spoon/actively attempts to clear
- ☐ Mouth opening
- ☐ Active lip movement
- ☐ Clears spoon
- ☐ Bolus propulsion
- ☐ Residue
- ☐ Cleans lips
- ☐ Tongue remains in mouth (no protrusion past incisors)
- ☐ Graded jaw movements
- ☐ Signs/symptoms of aspiration: ______________

Comments: ____

____

Chewables

Food(s) trialed: ____

____

Bite size: ____

____

Observations:
- ☐ Accepts food
- ☐ Lateralization
- ☐ Mastication
- ☐ Bolus formation/management
- ☐ Lip closure
- ☐ Food loss
- ☐ Bolus propulsion

- ☐ Vertical excursion (wide or small?)
- ☐ Initiates chew in timely manner
- ☐ Residue/management
- ☐ Sorting out textures
- ☐ Graded jaw movements (no associated head movement)
- ☐ Signs/symptoms of aspiration: ____________

Comments: ____

____

Biteables

Food(s) trialed: ____

____

Bite size: ____

____

Observations:
- ☐ Strength (lateral)
- ☐ Strength (anterior)
- ☐ Effectiveness
- ☐ Lips close around bolus
- ☐ Tongue remains retracted (not protruded beyond incisors, lips)
- ☐ Bolus formation/management
- ☐ Bolus propulsion
- ☐ Residue/management
- ☐ Signs/symptoms of aspiration: ____________

Comments: ____

____

Pharyngeal Concerns

☐ Delayed swallow	☐ Coughing	☐ Wet voice
☐ Multiple swallows	☐ Congestion	☐ Secretions
☐ Laryngeal elevation	☐ Other ____________	

PUTTING IT ALL TOGETHER

We have completed our assessment: We have historical information, observations of the child eating and drinking a wide variety of foods and liquids using a variety of utensils, and perhaps instrumental assessment results. Where are the results leading us as we attempt to move closer to the underlying cause (or causes) of the feeding and swallowing disorder? Our treatment plans will be built around the causative factors we've identified, keeping in mind that there's often more than one cause, of course. The following list provides an overview of some of those potential underlying problems as well as the assessment results that, together, indicate a specific cause.

Is it a respiratory problem?

- History of lung disease or early ventilator or oxygen dependence
- Coughing and choking with eating and drinking
- Impaired respiratory-swallow coordination
- Dyspnea
- Stress behaviors with feeding

Is it a GI problem?

- Frequent spit-up or vomiting
- Agitation or fussiness during and after feeds
- Poor sleep
- Constipation
- Loss of foods from repertoire
- Limited intake volume

Is it a sensory problem?

- Excessive gagging
- Specific preferences regarding utensils, textures, and temperatures
- Difficulty transitioning to new textures, tastes, temperatures, and utensils
- Less difficulty with liquids

- Separates "textured" portions of food and expels them
- Lack of mouth play or sensory seeking
- Restricted food repertoire
- Difficulty eating in new environments

Is it an oral motor problem?

- Difficulty with latch
- Drooling
- Limited tongue, lip, and jaw movement
- Speech difficulties
- Incoordination across textures
- Food loss out of mouth
- Difficulty learning to use new utensils
- Oral residue
- Accepts teething toys but is unable to bite or manipulate them

Is it a pharyngeal swallow problem?

- Abnormal cry and hoarse voice
- Stridor
- Coughing, choking, or sputtering
- Non-nutritive sucking better than nutritive sucking
- Drooling
- History of pulmonary illness
- Respiratory changes with feeding
- Instrumental assessment findings of swallow delay, pharyngeal dysmotility, or impaired airway protection

Now that we have an idea of what the problem is and what's causing it, let's put our treatment plan together!

3

What to Do When It's Breathing or Digestion—Or Both

Children can't (and won't) eat successfully if they're not comfortable. Unfortunately for many of our clients, physiological functions that should be pain free—and, in fact, imperceptible most of the time—are actually the source of considerable pain, pressure, and exertion. In this chapter, I'll explore respiratory and GI disorders, their impact on feeding and swallowing, and the medical interventions employed to treat them. Importantly, I will also discuss the feeding therapist's role in managing these disorders and identifying effective compensatory and therapeutic strategies.

RESPIRATION

Nothing matters if you can't breathe, right? That is certainly true for our clients. In fact, impairment in respiratory-swallow patterning is a common cause of feeding difficulties for many children on our caseloads. Babies born prematurely, children with respiratory disease, and children in need of tracheostomy or ventilatory support will all have potential difficulty coordinating breathing and swallowing.

Artificial Airways and Oxygen Delivery

Ventilators, tracheostomy, and noninvasive and invasive ventilation—the technology can be confusing. When it comes to breathing and respiration support, it is helpful to have an understanding of the technologies utilized to assist infants and children in maintaining oxygenation and ventilation.

Intubation and Ventilation

When babies and children are unable to breathe on their own, mechanical ventilation is used. Typically, an endotracheal (ET) tube is placed through the mouth, through the vocal folds, and into the trachea, allowing access to the lungs. A ventilator then provides oxygen and ventilation through the tube. Unfortunately, ET tubes can damage the larynx and put pressure on the palate, causing difficulties with feeding and swallowing once the client is extubated. For example, the persistent pressure of the tube on the palate can cause palate-pharyngeal incompetence and subsequent difficulty with nippling in infants when the tube is removed. Infants and children may also experience dysphagia symptoms post-extubation, including nasal regurgitation, breathing-swallow discoordination, and aspiration. This risk of dysphagia post-extubation increases with each hour of intubation (Hoffmeister et al., 2019).

Tracheostomy

When the need for artificial ventilation is prolonged, endotracheal intubation becomes impractical. Clients who are intubated must be sedated, and they are unable to communicate verbally or to receive nutrition orally. In these cases, conversion to tracheostomy is the next step. A surgeon creates a stoma, or opening, through the neck into the trachea, and a tracheostomy tube is placed in that stoma. The tracheostomy tube can then be connected to a ventilator if external ventilation is required. The presence of a tracheostomy tube creates a number of physiological changes—most notably, a change in expiratory airflow. Exhaled air no longer travels through the larynx, head, and neck. Instead, air moves in and out through the tracheostomy tube. This limits airflow through the larynx for voice and cough, and it limits airflow through the neck and head for smell and taste.

Infants and children with tracheostomy are far from a heterogenous group. Many have a variety of other medical conditions, including genetic conditions, pulmonary illnesses, neurological conditions, prematurity, and cardiac conditions, to name a few. Dysphagia is common in these clients, but it is sometimes difficult to determine if the dysphagia is the result of the tracheostomy tube itself or of the (often multiple) underlying conditions.

Noninvasive Positive Pressure Ventilation

Noninvasive positive pressure ventilation (NPPV) represents a significant step forward in the management of individuals who require mechanical ventilation, as it provides airway access without the need for endotracheal intubation. Instead, a facial mask is connected to a ventilator or BiPap unit that provides larger tidal volumes without an increase in respiratory effort. These airways have been demonstrated to reduce the need for intubation or re-intubation.

The relationship between noninvasive ventilation and swallowing has not been well-clarified in our literature as of yet. What we do know is that infants and children who require NPPV are fragile, with significant respiratory needs, and breathing-swallow coordination is likely to be compromised (Hirst et al., 2017). For example, individuals with muscular dystrophy have reported challenges in coordinating their breathing and swallowing when receiving NPPV, as well as difficulties in timing their chewing and swallowing with the breaths provided by the ventilator. However, most also reported less mealtime dyspnea and an increased ability to use cough to clear their airway (Britton et al., 2020).

High-Flow Nasal Cannula

High-flow nasal cannula (HFNC) allows for the provision of higher flow oxygen (as high as 60 liters per minute) through the use of a specialized nasal cannula. This eliminates the need for a facial mask, increases comfort, and allows for the provision of humidification. There is some evidence to suggest that HFNC may stimulate the respiratory center in premature infants and may decrease work of breathing (Mikalsen et al., 2016). As with NPPV, the relationship to swallowing disorders is unclear, and careful assessment of swallowing and respiration is critical.

Respiratory Diseases and Their Impact on Feeding and Swallowing

There are a number of respiratory diseases that feeding therapists encounter in their caseloads. The following are some of the more common disease processes and descriptions of what we know about their impact on feeding and swallowing.

Acute Respiratory Distress Syndrome

Acute respiratory distress syndrome (ARDS) is a condition that affects a number of infants born prematurely and is related to immature lung development, specifically to a lack of surfactant. Surfactant is a foamy fluid in the lungs that serves to keep the alveolar spaces open and available for gas exchange. Surfactant develops very near term and is often lacking in infants born before 34 weeks gestation. Without it, the alveoli collapse and work of breathing increases significantly. Infants with ARDS present with high respiratory rates, grunting and nasal flaring, chest retractions, apnea, and cyanosis. Babies with ARDS are often inefficient oral feeders due to their underlying respiratory compromise, prematurity, and medical instability.

Bronchopulmonary Dysplasia

While ARDS is an acute condition, bronchopulmonary dysplasia (BPD) is a chronic respiratory condition that comes about as a result of the respiratory interventions required in compromised infants, such as ventilation and high-flow oxygen therapy. These necessary, but high-pressure, interventions in immature lungs interfere with lung development, cause oxygen toxicity, and result in chronic disease. In extremely premature infants, BPD can result not only from the interventions themselves but also from very low birth weight and lack of alveolar surface area. Intubation trauma and laryngeal injury can accompany BPD and further compromise oral feeding potential. Infants with BPD typically present with suck-swallow-breathe discoordination, weak suckle pressures, high respiratory rates, and fatigue with feeding. Given the chronic nature of the condition, feeding difficulties may continue into childhood with persistent fatigue and impaired respiratory-swallow patterning.

Respiratory Syncytial Virus

Most of us have probably had respiratory syncytial virus, or RSV as it's more commonly known. In those of us with healthy lungs, it manifests as a cold with upper respiratory symptoms, but in infants and children with underlying lung disease, RSV can progress to a more severe condition with generalized inflammation of the respiratory tract, airway obstruction, apnea, and pneumonia. Aspiration risk increases in babies and children with RSV bronchiolitis due to low tolerance for swallow apnea and disordered respiratory-swallow coordination (Khoshoo & Edell, 1999; Pinnington et al., 2000).

COVID-19

Given the recency of the onset of the COVID-19 virus, there is scarce evidence regarding its impact on feeding and swallowing. Children seem to be impacted by the virus at a significantly lower frequency than adults, and when they are infected, they typically have milder symptoms. A small percentage of children, however, have had serious respiratory complications as a result of COVID-19, and children with pre-existing comorbidities have been disproportionately impacted. Children with tracheostomy and other pulmonary conditions in particular are at higher risk (Shekerdemian et al., 2020). Anecdotal information (and my own personal experience in treating COVID patients) suggests that laryngeal trauma post-extubation, impaired breathing-swallow coordination, and generalized weakness are contributing to increased aspiration risk in this fragile group of patients.

Compensatory Strategies

So when the problem is breathing, what can we do? In these cases, we can apply a variety of compensatory strategies, including bolus manipulation, external pacing, and bolus holding.

Bolus Manipulation

There is a great deal of variability in the swallow response. The onset of the swallow, the degree of tongue-base retraction, the onset and duration of laryngeal closure, and the onset and duration of the upper esophageal sphincter all change from swallow to swallow, depending in large part on the sensory characteristics of the bolus. Therefore, we can manipulate the characteristics of the bolus to facilitate improvements in respiratory-swallow patterning. The following are two bolus characteristics to consider modifying:

- **Bolus size:** Not surprisingly, larger boluses result in earlier onset and longer duration of laryngeal valve closure to ensure adequate airway protection (Hiss et al., 2001). We can turn that to our advantage and utilize smaller boluses with babies and children who are having difficulty with breathing-swallow coordination or dyspnea with eating. Smaller boluses mean later onset of breathing cessation and more time for breathing.

- **Flow rate:** Similar to reducing the bolus size, slowing the flow rate decreases the demands on the respiratory system (Chang et al., 2007). Choose a nipple with a slower flow for infants or a covered cup that allows for flow control for children. However, a change in flow rate or utensil requires a degree of motor adaptation, so the baby or child must be given adequate time to adjust to the new rate before we can judge its effectiveness.

  Breastfeeding mothers can reduce the flow of their breastmilk by briefly occluding some ducts by pressing on them with the side of their hand during breastfeeding. Care should be taken to occlude the ducts only briefly and to change the hand position to avoid continuous occlusion of the same ducts. In addition, you should involve lactation consultants when considering these types of interventions. Pumping breastmilk during the letdown (before placing the baby at the breast) can also be helpful in avoiding the high flow associated with the letdown, but it should be done sparingly, as this practice may reduce the mother's milk supply. Breast pumps do not empty the breasts with the same efficiency that a baby can and, over time, can result in reductions in milk supply among women who pump extensively. You can also use thickeners to slow the flow rate of liquids, but this intervention brings with it a number of potential complications. (See chapter 4 for a full discussion of the pros and cons of thickening.)

External Pacing

Imposing breaks on the infant or child while eating or drinking can also be an effective tool for reducing the demands that swallowing places on the respiratory system (Dozier et al., 2006). With infants, pause the feeding when the infant appears to be having difficulty with respiratory-swallow patterning or dyspnea. Encourage single sips rather than serial swallows for children. See chapter 2 for a full description of the stress behaviors to watch for. We can help children pace themselves by alternating between easy-to-chew foods and hard-to-chew foods, or by alternating between bites of food and sips of liquid. Below is an example of how to place foods on a plate to encourage pacing. The chicken requires more chewing, so it is alternated with yogurt to provide the child with a break from chewing.

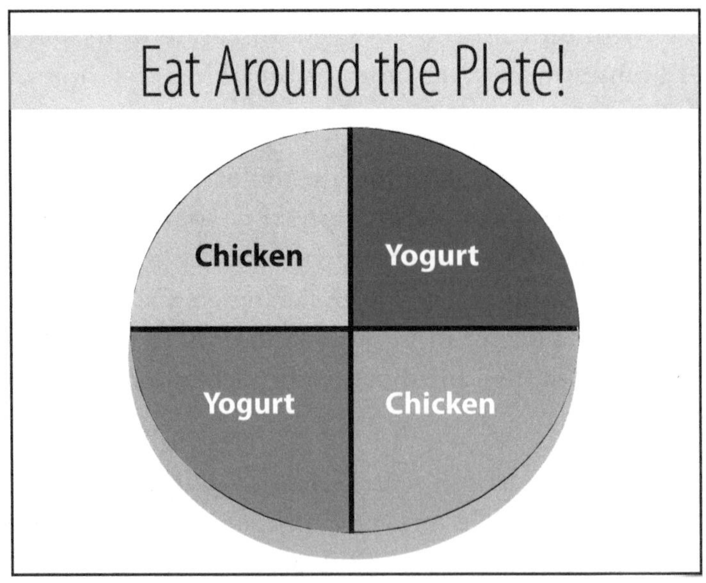

Bolus Holding

As children get older, we can teach them to voluntarily impact their respiratory-swallow patterning by using a bolus "hold," which is a technique that has been well-established in adult patient populations (Curtis & Troche, 2020; Martin-Harris et al., 2015). Instruct the child to take a sip of liquid, to take a bite of puree, or to chew their higher-texture food—but just before the swallow, to stop for a second and then swallow. This technique helps regulate breathing and can facilitate more consistent use of a post-swallow exhalation pattern. By tapping into the *voluntary* components of the swallow response, we may also be improving oral containment and thereby reducing any pre-swallow entry of the bolus into the pharynx. You can use the client handout on the next page to teach bolus holding to children.

Client Handout

Learning the Bolus Hold Technique

Sometimes we run out of air when we try to eat. Whenever you eat, try this technique to make it easier to breathe AND eat.

1. Take a bite

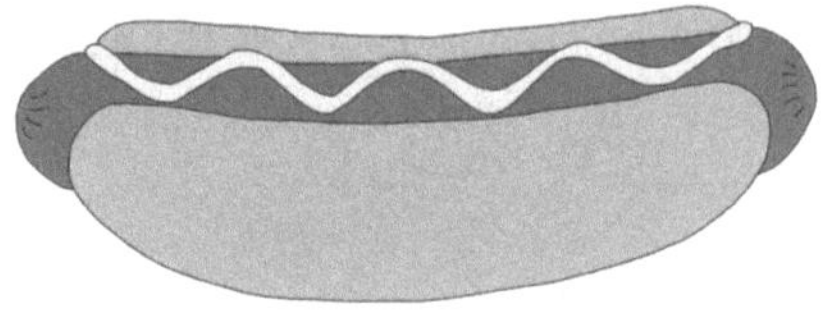

2. CHEW CHEW CHEW

3. STOP

4. Swallow!

5. Breathe out

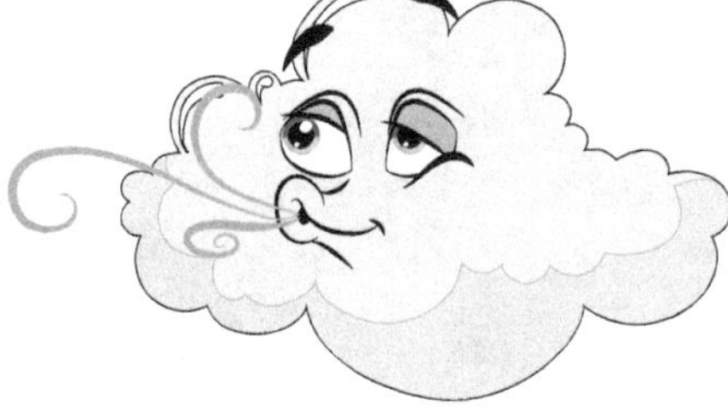

Interventions

In addition to the previous compensatory strategies, you can use the following interventions when problems with respiration are contributing to feeding and swallowing difficulties.

Non-Nutritive Sucking

There is a growing body of research to support non-nutritive sucking, or pacifier use, with infants. Non-nutritive sucking improves state regulation and overall readiness for oral feeding, decreases length of NICU stay, facilitates transition from tube feeding to nippling, and results in better bottle-feeding performance (Foster et al., 2016). Non-nutritive sucking may also improve respiratory-swallow patterning and suck-swallow-breathe coordination, but this may be less of a direct impact and more the result of improvements in state regulation. A calmer baby can certainly breathe better!

Oral Stimulation

Research has demonstrated that oral interventions—specifically those that provide sensory stimulation to the cheeks, lips, and jaw; intraoral stimulation to the inside of the mouth; and non-nutritive sucking—have the potential to improve respiratory-swallow patterning in preterm infants (Fucile et al., 2012). It seems, then, that providing positive, pleasurable sensory input can regulate breathing and have a positive impact on breathing-swallow coordination. However, be sure that the stimulation is in fact pleasurable. And never force your way into a baby's mouth. Gently touching the child's philtrum, lips, or cheeks can stimulate a mouth-opening response. Wait for that response before attempting any intraoral stimulation.

Expiratory Muscle Strength Training

Therapists have long understood the importance of building core stability and strength. Better core strength results in better upper and lower extremity function, better head and neck control, and even better oral motor function. We also know that the respiratory muscles are an important subset of the muscles that make up the core. Consequently, a client with respiratory muscle weakness likely has core weakness, and a client with core weakness likely has respiratory muscle weakness.

But can we specifically target the respiratory muscle portion of the core to improve breathing function—and subsequently breathing-swallow coordination? It appears that we can through expiratory muscle strength training (EMST). With this intervention, clients forcefully blow through an EMST device and meet resistance provided through a one-way spring-loaded valve. That resistance is calibrated and can be continually increased to increase the demand on the muscles. Through this progressive resistance, we can increase respiratory muscle strength and function, improve cough response and airway protection, and improve breathing-swallow coordination.

There is a great deal of evidence to support this therapeutic technique with adult clients of various disabilities, including chronic obstructive pulmonary disease, cerebrovascular accidents, and other neuromuscular diseases. While there are fewer research studies involving pediatric clients, the existing research suggests that EMST is effective for children as well (Cerny et al., 1997). However, given the muscular effort and degree of voluntary control required, the exercise is not appropriate for children under five years of age.

Positioning

We know that inefficiencies in respiration can result from weakness in the respiratory musculature. We can compensate for these inefficiencies at least in part through changes in positioning. Upright, stable positioning with a good base of support for the feet can improve trunk stability and respiratory support. For infants, elevated side-lying can be helpful in facilitating optimal suck-swallow-breathe coordination.

Improving Respiratory Control

Breathing and swallowing are similar functions in that they both have reflexive properties. However, they are also both functions over which we can exert voluntary control, and there is therapeutic value in assigning activities to children that provide them with that voluntary control over their breathing. Virtually any activity that involves breathing can help provide that control. Whether it's focusing on inhaling versus exhaling, holding our breath, letting the breath out slowly, letting the breath out quickly, taking big breaths, or taking little breaths, these activities can all provide children with more awareness of their own breathing and, in turn, help them develop greater control. Try some of these activities while manipulating the volume of the breath and the speed of the exhalation:

- **Blowing bubbles:** A fast exhalation will result in lots of little bubbles, while a slow exhalation will create one larger bubble.
- **Blowing a pinwheel:** Can the child make the wheel spin fast? Slow?

- **Blowing whistles or horns:** Can the child use their breath to make a loud sound? A soft sound? Can they make one long sound? Several short sounds?
- **Blowing cotton balls or ping-pong balls across the table:** Can the child make them go fast? Slow? Can they blow them only partway across the table? Can they blow them completely off the table?
- **Singing:** Can the child make their voice really loud? Very soft? Can they take a big breath and hold the note for a few seconds?

Virtually any activity you can think of that involves breathing will work.

GASTROINTESTINAL FUNCTION AND DYSFUNCTION

Gastrointestinal Disorders and Their Impact on Feeding and Swallowing

We've already established that one of the most common causes of food refusal in children is GI dysfunction. To put it simply, children won't eat if they don't feel well. In this section, you'll find a list of GI disorders that feeding therapists are likely to encounter and a description of their impact on feeding and swallowing.

Gastroesophageal Reflux Disease

Everybody has reflux episodes; they are a normal part of gastric functioning. However, the term *gastroesophageal reflux disease*, or GERD, is reserved for reflux that is excessive and that results in physiological issues and medical problems. The signs and symptoms of GERD are variable in that the same child can have one set of symptoms today and a different set of symptoms next week. Some of the more common symptoms of GERD in babies and children include limitations in repertoire, low volume of intake, loss of previously consumed foods, food refusal, and discomfort and irritability during eating. Chapter 2 contains a more exhaustive list of the many signs and symptoms of GERD in babies and children, including esophageal, pulmonary, oral, and ear, nose, and throat symptoms (see the section on "Gastrointestinal Function").

Feeding Behaviors Associated with GERD

Infants:

- Food refusal
- Arched back, turned away from nipple
- Food aversions, selectivity
- Coughing or choking
- Hiccups
- Irritability
- Vomiting

Children:

- Food refusal
- Loss of foods from repertoire
- Low intake volume
- Abdominal pain
- Burping or belching
- Choking, gagging
- Difficulty swallowing
- Pain with swallowing

Babies and children with underlying GI issues clearly require medical intervention and oversight. However, there are some interventions that feeding and swallowing therapists can help with, which can involve making dietary modifications, increasing saliva, making lifestyle modifications, and facilitating eubiosis. When this is not enough, medications and medical management may become necessary.

Dietary Modifications

For formula-fed babies experiencing reflux, physicians will often recommend changing to a soy-based formula or, in more severe cases, to an extensively hydrolyzed protein formula. Added-rice formulas can also be effective in reducing reflux, but these formulas often have cow's milk protein as an ingredient and are therefore not effective if the underlying issue is a cow's milk protein intolerance or allergy. Although there is a long-standing practice of thickening formula with baby cereal to manage reflux, research has demonstrated that this practice does not have an impact on the *number* of reflux episodes and only impacts the *height* of the regurgitation (Rosen et al., 2018). If the infant is in danger of aspirating the refluxed material, then reducing the number of full-column reflux episodes can reduce that risk. For breastfed babies, modifications to the mother's diet are often suggested. For example, reducing or eliminating dairy and hens' eggs may be helpful in reducing excessive reflux in these babies.

As babies move into the toddler years and beyond, it is important to identify the foods that trigger reflux episodes or other periods of gut discomfort. Dairy and wheat are often implicated in GI pathologies, but any food allergen can potentially cause reflux episodes, diarrhea, constipation, and vomiting. In addition, we know that we can sometimes improve symptoms by adding foods that are more easily digested, such as proteins and simple carbohydrates. Adding fluid and fiber to the diet can also be helpful in reducing constipation and the reflux episodes that often accompany it.

The Importance of Saliva

Saliva is an important bodily fluid with a number of physiological roles. It lubricates the oral structures to facilitate movement for speech, chewing, and bolus manipulation; it initiates the digestive process by breaking down starches; it helps maintain oral health by managing bacteria; and it helps manage reflux. Because our saliva acts as a natural antacid, when we swallow saliva, it serves to neutralize acid in the esophagus and stomach—and the mechanical act of swallowing saliva results in an esophageal peristaltic wave that further facilitates esophageal clearance.

Therefore, increasing saliva swallows can be a helpful tool in the management of excessive acidic reflux. For babies and young children, you can increase saliva swallows by encouraging non-nutritive sucking on a pacifier or toy. For children with sufficient oral motor skills, gum chewing can be effective in increasing saliva production and, in turn, saliva swallows.

Lifestyle Modifications

There is a direct link between stress and excessive reflux, which is related to blood flow and the fight-or-flight response. When we are under stress, either perceived or actual, our sympathetic nervous system responds by secreting stress hormones, including epinephrine and norepinephrine. This hormonal secretion has a number of effects on the body, including increased heart rate, increased blood pressure, increased blood sugar levels, and blood flow shift. Through the varying constriction and dilation of blood vessels, blood flow is shifted away from digestion and toward muscles responsible for fighting or fleeing. As a result, digestion slows or stops, which has the effect of increasing the likelihood of reflux episodes.

Therefore, reducing stress responses in our clients can be an effective tool for reducing reflux episodes. We can inhibit the fight-or-flight response and normalize digestive functioning in children by making mealtimes fun and creating positive associations around eating and food. Chapter 6 provides detailed suggestions to reduce anxiety around eating and increase participation.

Other lifestyle changes include increasing the time between the last meal of the day and sleep. In other words, go to bed on an empty (or a near-empty) stomach to reduce nighttime reflux episodes. Even those of us without reflux disease are more susceptible to reflux episodes at night because when we are sleeping, we are in a reclined position, and the tone in both the upper and lower esophageal sphincters is somewhat reduced. Nighttime reflux episodes are particularly problematic for babies and children with reflux disease, and families should seek guidance from their pediatricians regarding safe sleep positions. Generally, the recommendation is supine but elevated for infants, and either supine and elevated or side-lying and elevated for children. Finally, limiting exposure to secondhand smoke can help reduce symptoms in infants and children given that nicotine (even through secondhand exposure) lowers the tone in the lower esophageal sphincter.

Facilitating Eubiosis

We have established the importance of the gut microbiome in developing the immune system, protecting against pathogens, and facilitating digestion. However, there are a variety of unavoidable and necessary interventions that have a negative impact on the microbiome, including antibiotics, proton-pump inhibitors, tube feeding, and mechanical ventilation. Stress can impact the gut microbiome too. But can we be proactive? Are there ways to impact the development and maintenance of the microbiome in a positive manner to create a diverse, balanced bacterial environment? Research indicates that there are some evidence-based interventions that can help (Dunlop et al., 2015; Milani et al., 2017):

- **Skin-to-skin care** allows babies to acquire more of their parents' skin microbiome and less of the hospital microbiome on blankets, sheets, and medical equipment.
- **Breastfeeding** or bottle-feeding with fresh breastmilk facilitates gut development and the creation of a healthy microbiome and immune system.
- **Probiotics and prebiotics** are being used with increasing frequency for the management of GI issues and have been shown to decrease the number of infections, decrease fussiness and crying associated with

colic, and decrease antibiotic-associated diarrhea. Probiotics are live microbial cells that are often added to formula and foods to establish healthy flora colonization. They have proven to be helpful in decreasing regurgitation and improving gastric motility (Indrio et al., 2017; Milani et al., 2017). Probiotics can be found naturally in soy products, pickled vegetables, kombucha, and fermented dairy products, including yogurt, buttermilk, and kefir.

Probiotics are sometimes combined with prebiotics, or nondigestible carbohydrates, which stimulate bacterial growth. Prebiotics can be found naturally in a number of foods—including garlic, raw leeks, raw onion, wheat flour, and bananas—and are available as supplements as well. While probiotics and prebiotics occur naturally in many foods, are largely available over the counter, and are generally thought to be safe, they can have adverse effects in preterm infants and those with immune deficiencies, irritable bowel syndrome, and short bowel syndrome. Therefore, they should always be taken under the supervision of the child's pediatrician or gastroenterologist.

Medications and Medical Interventions

If dietary and lifestyle modifications are not effective on their own in alleviating reflux, physicians may consider medical interventions, including medications or, in intractable cases, surgery. As feeding therapists, we are clearly not in the position to prescribe medications or order procedures, but it is still helpful to have an understanding of the medications our clients are taking and the procedures they may undergo.

There are five categories of medication utilized for the management of GERD symptoms: antacids, physical barriers, prokinetics, histamine blockers, and proton-pump inhibitors. Although these medications are useful in alleviating the symptoms of reflux, they also carry a variety of side effects associated with acid suppression. Stomach acids are important to digestion, maintenance of the microbiome, and immune system functioning, and alterations to the gastric environment through the use of histamine blockers or proton-pump inhibitors can have undesirable effects.

For example, acid suppression has been linked to a variety of nutritional deficiencies, including anemia, impaired B-12 absorption, and impaired calcium absorption. There also have been documented instances of bacterial overgrowth as a result of acid suppression, which can result in increased infections, including community-acquired pneumonia, enterocolitis, and gastroenteritis.

You can find a full review of the evidence and recommendations regarding proton-pump inhibitor use in children in the Pediatric Gastroesophageal Reflux Clinical Practice Guidelines (Rosen et al., 2018).

Medication	Mechanism	Examples	Availability and Use
Antacids	Neutralize acids after their production	Tums®, Rolaids®	• Over the counter • Generally not utilized with pediatric clients
Physical barriers	Coat stomach and create a protective barrier	Gaviscon®, Pepto-Bismol®	• Over the counter • Gaviscon is available in prescription strength
Prokinetics	Speed up stomach emptying	Reglan®	• Prescription only • Recommended for short-term use only due to significant risk of side effects
Histamine blockers (aka H_2 receptor agonists)	Slow acid production at the cellular level by inhibiting action of histamines	Zantac®, Pepcid®	• Available over the counter but generally by prescription for pediatric clients
Proton-pump inhibitors	Significantly suppress acid via inhibition of the proton pumps within stomach cells	Prevacid® Prilosec®	• Available over the counter but generally by prescription for pediatric clients • Utilized in the treatment of erosive disease • Have been linked to nutritional deficiencies and increased risk of infection

When all other options have been exhausted, physicians may consider a surgical option for the treatment of GERD: the fundoplication. During the procedure, the surgeon wraps the fundus, or upper vestibule of the stomach, around the lower esophageal sphincter to reinforce that sphincter. This procedure can be an effective tool for the management of severe reflux disease, but given that it disrupts pressure within the digestive system, it has the potential to result in retching, gas, bloating, and early entry of stomach contents into the duodenum and intestine, particularly in infants and young children whose digestive systems are still developing.

Constipation

Sometimes, it's all about the poop. Constipation is a common cause of food refusal in children. Infrequent bowel movements result in a "backup" to the system, which causes pain and discomfort, early satiety, and increased frequency and severity of reflux episodes. Given the variability in the frequency of bowel movements in infants and children, there is disagreement about how exactly to define constipation. Physicians would generally agree, however, that bowel movements that occur less than three times per week, are hard and difficult to pass, cause pain, or are bloody would be abnormal. Helping children poop on a regular basis can normalize digestive functions and improve readiness for feeding.

Adding fluid and fiber to the child's diet are generally first-line interventions for the management of constipation. Pear and prune juice, plenty of fresh fruits and vegetables, beans and legumes, and high-fiber cereals can help normalize bowel function. As previously discussed, yogurt and other fermented dairy products contain natural probiotics that can be an additional tool for managing constipation. If you are working with a child to address issues related to pharyngeal dysphagia in addition to constipation, take care when implementing dietary modifications, as some interventions used to manage aspiration risk can limit access to fluid and fiber (see chapter 4).

To normalize bowel movements, it can also be useful to assist the family in implementing a regular toileting schedule. Encourage toileting at a similar time each day, and provide any needed assistance to position the child on the toilet in order to facilitate normal stooling patterns.

Finally, stool softeners are often employed when dietary modifications are insufficient to normalize bowel functions. Stimulant laxatives, enemas, and manual disimpaction are generally prescribed only when other options have failed.

Food Allergies

For reasons that are not well understood, food allergies in children are increasing dramatically (Jackson et al., 2013). Some researchers attribute this to the overuse of antibiotics and acid-suppressing medications. Others adhere to the "hygiene hypothesis," which suggests that our overreliance on germ-killing, antimicrobial cleaners has made us more susceptible to allergens. Regardless of the underlying reason behind this increase, food allergies represent an additional consideration when working with children with gastric dysfunction who present with issues related to food refusal and limitations in food repertoire.

In order to understand food allergies, we must first discuss immunoglobulin E, which is a blood antibody that is released into the bloodstream in response to an allergen. Some allergens trigger the release of the antibody and are referred to as IgE-mediated allergies, whereas others do not trigger its release and are referred to as non-IgE-mediated allergies (or "intolerances"). Food allergies can be either IgE-mediated or non-IgE-mediated.

IgE versus Non-IgE Food Allergies

IgE-mediated food allergies:

- Produce immediate reactions
- Cause reactions that are often severe (e.g., anaphylaxis, vomiting)
- Can be identified via blood tests

Non-IgE-mediated food allergies:

- Produce delayed reactions, sometimes days after the allergen is ingested
- Are not easily identified by blood tests and require food challenge testing
- Are more likely to affect the GI system

The gastric discomfort associated with food allergies or intolerances can result in food refusal, limitations in food repertoire, coughing, gagging, laryngeal and pharyngeal swelling and inflammation, and increased mucus production throughout the entire aerodigestive tract. Children with food allergies often present with delays in oral motor development as well, resulting from a lack of practice with a variety of foods and utensils.

Eosinophilic Esophagitis

Eosinophilic esophagitis (EoE) is an inflammatory condition caused by food allergies in which eosinophils, which are a type of white blood cell, increase in number in the esophageal wall. Symptoms mimic reflux disease and, in fact, EoE and GERD sometimes co-occur. Like GERD and food allergies, EoE can cause food refusals, low intake volume, prolonged feeding times, and limitations in food repertoire. Failure to transition to textured food, delays in oral motor skill development, gagging, vomiting, and failure to thrive have also been associated with EoE. This condition is diagnosed via endoscopic biopsy. Once diagnosed, treatments may include elemental or hypoallergenic formulas and food elimination diets.

Formulas Used with Food Allergies and Intolerances

Partially Hydrolyzed	Extensively Hydrolyzed	Amino Acid-Based
• These are not hypoallergenic but can help with GERD not related to the allergy • Examples: Gerber® Good Start®, Enfamil™ Gentlease®	• These are largely hypoallergenic, but some infants may still react since they may contain cow's milk protein • Examples: Similac® Alimentum®, Nutramigen™, Pregestimil®	• These are hypoallergenic formulas • Examples: Neocate®, EleCare®, Nutramigen® AA

Children with known or suspected food allergies or EoE require ongoing medical assessment and management by a gastroenterologist or an allergist. Once we have assurance that the allergies are well managed, we may need to employ behavioral techniques to free children from the anxiety and learned food avoidance (see chapter 6).

IS IT BREATHING, DIGESTION, OR BOTH?

As discussed in chapter 1, breathing and digestion are interrelated functions, and we have established that dysfunction in either system can cause deficits in feeding and swallowing. There are also several disease processes that can potentially cause dysfunction in all three systems: breathing, digestion, and swallowing.

Asthma is a chronic respiratory disease that results in inflammation and bronchial narrowing, which makes it difficult to breathe. In some individuals with asthma, there is a potential GERD and dysphagia component as well.

That's because both the respiratory and GI systems are innervated by the vagus nerve, so any interruption in the vagal response can result in symptoms in both systems. For example, a vagal response originating in the esophagus that is triggered by a reflux episode can cause a respiratory response that may include bronchial constriction and worsening of asthma. Extraesophageal reflux (EER), or reflux that comes through the esophagus and enters the pharynx, can also result in many ear, nose, and throat symptoms. If aspiration of acidic reflux occurs, even in microscopic amounts, bronchial inflammation, airway constriction, and mucus overproduction can result, exacerbating asthma attacks and making the asthma much harder to control.

There are other interactions between the breathing and digestive systems that manifest themselves in clients with asthma and GERD. For example, the chronic cough associated with asthma can cause a diaphragmatic contraction that forces stomach contents into the esophagus. The increased work of breathing associated with asthma exacerbations can also pull energy from the GI system and slow gastric emptying, which then results in a higher likelihood of reflux episodes occurring. In addition, asthma medications (known as bronchodilators) lower the tone in the lower esophageal sphincter and increase reflux episodes. Therefore, if one of your client's comorbidities is asthma, be on the lookout for the signs and symptoms of feeding disorders associated with GERD, including food refusals and limitations in repertoire.

Laryngomalacia is a condition in which the laryngeal cartilages above the vocal folds collapse, resulting in stridor. The stridor is worse when the baby is in a supine position, is crying, or is feeding. The cause, or more likely causes, of laryngomalacia include immature tissue, underlying neurological deficits, and hypotonia. The resulting increase in work of breathing, potential for decreased laryngeal sensation, and difficulty with suck-swallow-breathe coordination often result in pharyngeal dysphagia and feeding difficulties, including coughing, choking, and worsening of stridor during feedings.

GERD often co-exists with laryngomalacia, though a direct causal relationship between these conditions has not been established. Laryngomalacia impacts intrathoracic pressure, which can exacerbate reflux. The resulting acid exposure to the airway appears to cause swelling of laryngeal tissues, which then exacerbates airway collapse. However, it's unclear what exactly causes what. What we do know is that managing GERD symptoms can result in improvement in stridor and decrease swelling and tissue collapse. In addition to medical management of their GERD, clients with laryngomalacia will benefit from many of the compensatory strategies discussed earlier in this chapter to improve breathing-swallow coordination and to decrease work of breathing during feedings.

Finally, *obstructive sleep apnea (OSA)* is characterized by apnea, or breathing cessation, during sleep and is caused by partial or complete upper airway collapse. It often co-occurs with GERD for reasons that are not well understood. Pressure changes in the lungs associated with the apneic episodes have been hypothesized to force stomach contents into the esophagus, triggering reflux episodes. Increased work of breathing following an apneic episode may also contribute to lower esophageal sphincter relaxation and reflux episodes. An alternate theory is that the reflux is the trigger for the apnea, such that the acidic refluxate in the esophagus and pharynx causes the airway collapse and subsequent apneic episode. Delays in swallow response have been identified in individuals with OSA, but whether this is linked to the GERD or to a separate mechanism is not clear. Clients with OSA should be evaluated for changes in pharyngeal swallow function and should be monitored for signs and symptoms of GERD as well.

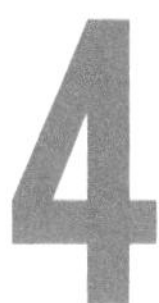

Guzzle, Gobble, and Gulp: Pharyngeal Swallow Management

Pediatric clients with pharyngeal dysphagia are a high-risk group of children. Pharyngeal dysphagia can result in a number of adverse health consequences, including aspiration, lung disease, respiratory infections, malnutrition, and dehydration. When children with this disorder aspirate, the pulmonary consequences can be immediately apparent (e.g., chronic cough, shortness of breath, respiratory infection) or present over the long term (e.g., lung scarring and chronic lung disease).

Management of pharyngeal dysphagia and its potential health consequences requires intervention that occurs on a number of different fronts, which may include reduction of risk through diet management, compensations and oral hygiene interventions, and therapeutic interventions to improve swallow function over time.

DIET MANAGEMENT STRATEGIES

Our first line of defense as we manage known or potential aspiration risk is typically diet management. Unfortunately, there has historically not been consistency in either terminology or implementation of various diet levels. To remedy this concern, an international group of clinicians recently came together to standardize our approach to dietary modifications (Steele et al., 2018). The result was the International Dysphagia Diet Standardization Initiative (IDDSI), which provides global standards for labeling texture-modified foods and thickened liquids.* Using those standards, the following

* Be sure to check out https://iddsi.org for detailed descriptions and information about testing procedures to aid in identification of viscosity and texture.

table provides definitions of some common terms when working with individuals with swallowing difficulties.

Food Type	Description	Examples
Pureed foods	• Do not require chewing • Too thick to be poured (will not flow from a cup) • Do not contain lumps • Cohesive (liquid portion does not separate and holds shape on a plate)	Infant cereals, some commercial baby foods, puddings, blenderized meats and vegetables, yogurt (without fruit chunks)
Minced and moist foods	• Do not require biting • Minimal chewing required • Soft and moist • May have visible lumps that are easily mashed by the tongue	Chopped meats, mashed fruits or vegetables, oatmeal
Soft and bite-sized foods	• Require chewing but not biting • Can be mashed with fork or other utensil • Soft throughout (no hard lumps)	Soft cooked meats in small pieces, soft fruits or vegetables in small pieces
Easy-to-chew foods	• Require chewing and some biting • Textured but not stringy or fibrous • Can be cut with a fork	Tender meats, cooked vegetables, most fruits
Regular foods	• No restrictions • May include foods that are hard, chewy, or fibrous • Include mixed-texture foods	Raw vegetables, all meats, all fruits, nuts or seeds, soups or stews
Liquid Type	**Description**	**Examples**
Extremely thick	• Same as puree	Same as puree
Moderately thick	• Thick but will drip from a fork in dollops	"Runny" baby foods, some yogurt drinks or smoothies
Mildly thick	• Slower than thin drinks but flows easily from a spoon	Some yogurt drinks, some infant formulas
Thin	• Fast flow	Water, broth, juice, milk

Using these standards, we can make recommendations for the texture of the food and the viscosity of the liquids in order to reduce choking risk and aspiration. But what are the appropriate diet interventions? Before choosing a "safe" diet, we have to identify the specific impairment (or impairments) causing the dysphagia. What did your clinical and instrumental assessments reveal as the causative factors? Let that information guide your diet choices.

When to Thicken

Because thickening slows the flow of liquid and makes it easier to control (Newman et al., 2016), it can be an effective compensation when the following impairments are present:

- Impaired oral bolus control
- Impaired breathing-swallow coordination
- Delayed swallow response
- Delayed or incomplete laryngeal closure or elevation

Thicker liquids, however, are heavier and require more "work" in some cases (Frazier & Friedman, 1996; Sia et al., 2018). Thickening, then, would *not* be an effective compensation when the underlying impairments include:

- Impaired tongue propulsion
- Impaired pharyngeal motility or "squeeze"

The following table provides some different examples of thickener types, as well as the mechanism by which they work and their benefits and limitations.

Thickener Type	Thickening Mechanism	Advantages	Disadvantages	Examples
Starch	Absorption (starch molecules absorb liquid to thicken)	• Easily mixed by hand • Adds calories	• Slow to thicken and continues to thicken over time • Added starch may be problematic for clients with diabetes • Can cause loose stools • Adds cost to care	Thick-It® Thick & Easy®
Gum/gel	Bonding (gum molecules bond to each other to thicken)	• Thickens quickly and maintains stability over time	• Can be difficult to mix • Xanthan gum is linked to necrotizing enterocolitis in premature infants and is not approved for children under 12 months of age • Adds cost to care	Simply Thick® ThickenUp Clear®
Baby cereals	Absorption	• Inexpensive • Readily available	• Lack of stability (separates quickly) • Imprecise (difficult to achieve consistency) • Adds considerable number of calories and can be difficult to digest for infants • Constipating	Infant rice cereal Infant oatmeal

Thickener Type	Thickening Mechanism	Advantages	Disadvantages	Examples
Carob bean/ locust bean gum	Bonding (as with other gum products)	• Mixes easily	• Adds cost to care (often more expensive than other products) • Thickens slowly over time • Must use with warm liquids • Approved for use with infants only after 42 weeks of gestation	Gelmix™
Food products	Absorption	• Readily available • Inexpensive	• Difficult to maintain consistency • Often thickens unevenly and separates • Significantly alters taste of liquid • Potentially adds sugar, fat, and additional calories	Banana flakes Potato flakes Corn starch Instant pudding
Pre-thickened liquids	N/A	• Ease of use • Reduced caregiver burden	• Adds cost to care (often more expensive than other products) • Limited to water, juice, and milk in most product lines	Thick & Easy Thick-It Clear Advantage™

When to Modify Food Texture

Softer, more cohesive foods are easier to manage for some children, as they require little to no biting or chewing. They can be used to compensate for the following impairments:

- Impaired oral bolus control
- Impaired mastication
- Reduced jaw strength or impaired bite
- Fatigue with chewing
- Impulsivity or increased rate of intake with insufficient mastication

When determining appropriate and safe food textures, consider the child's oral motor skills and match them to the food types. You can use the following table as a guide.

Type of Food	Oral Motor Skills Required
Pureed foods	• Emerging anterior-posterior tongue movement • Emerging lip closure • Emerging upper lip movement
Minced/moist foods	• Anterior-posterior tongue movement • Emerging vertical jaw movement • Emerging tongue-body lateralization • Tongue/jaw differentiation • Emerging bite
Soft, bite-sized foods	• Persistent vertical jaw movement • Tongue-body lateralization • Emerging tongue-tip lateralization • Jaw stability • Emerging bite
Easy-to-chew foods	• Persistent vertical jaw movement • Emerging rotary jaw movement • Full tongue lateralization • Jaw stability • Emerging bite • Lip/tongue differentiation
Regular solids	• Rotary jaw movement • Internal jaw stability • Full lip/tongue/jaw differentiation • Full tongue lateralization • Consistent bite

In addition to the IDDSI classifications, we can consider "dissolvable" or "meltable" solids for children who are having difficulty making the transition from pureed to solid foods. These are foods that quickly dissolve to puree in the mouth with minimal to no chewing or bolus manipulation. Examples include baby puffs, veggie or yogurt "melts," and Cheerios™.

Consequences of Dietary Modifications

Although it is tempting to think about dietary changes as being fairly benign interventions, we need to think carefully when deciding to make modifications. The fact is, when you modify a person's diet, you need to weigh the consequences of doing so against the benefits of the potential change. Let's consider some of the consequences of food texture changes.

Developmental Issues

Consider your long-term goal: Are you expecting that this child will move on to manage higher-texture foods or thinner liquids? If so, then they are going to have to practice. (See chapter 5 for a full discussion of oral motor learning techniques.) Modified diets are very effective at compensating for deficits in pharyngeal swallow function, but they do not provide opportunities for motor learning or skill development. If the goal is to help the client develop a more advanced diet, then we have to include opportunities for practice in our treatment plan.

Nutrition

We can achieve lower textures, like puree and minced and moist foods, by adding fluids to the food item. While these fluids bring texture down and increase cohesion and smoothness, they also have the potential to dilute caloric and protein density and to reduce flavor intensity. It is difficult, then, to provide sufficient calories and protein on commercially available pureed "baby food." Families will have to prepare their own pureed or soft foods and will need assistance with recipes, food preparation, and strategies to maintain nutritional variety. The following handout contains resources for parents and clinicians to help with pureed food preparation.

Client Handout

Resources for Families: Pureed Food Preparation

When your child needs a special diet, it can be challenging to find or prepare the appropriate foods. Here are some websites, cookbooks, and recipes that can help.

Websites

- www.essentialpuree.com
- You can also check out the Muscular Dystrophy Association, which has suggestions for "easy swallowing" foods: https://www.mda.org/quest/article/i-can-eat-cookbook-easy-chewing-and-swallowing

Cookbooks

- *Easy-to-Swallow, Easy-to-Chew Cookbook* by Donna Weihofen, JoAnne Robbins, and Paula Sullivan (2002)
- *Essential Purée: The A to Z Guidebook* by Diane Wolff (2016)
- *Soft Foods for Easier Eating Cookbook* by Sandra Woodruff and Leah Gilbert-Henderson (2007)
- *The Dysphagia Cookbook* by Elayne Achilles (2004)
- *The I-Can't-Chew Cookbook* by J. Randy Wilson (2003)
- *The Purées of Spring* by Diane Wolff (2020)
- *Think Outside the Blender* by Maria Quici (2014)

Products

Check out these solid foods that melt to puree in your mouth:

- EAT Bars™ (www.theeatbar.com)
- Savorease™ products (www.savorease.com)

There are also companies that sell prepared gourmet puree:

- Gourmet Puréed (www.gourmetpureed.com)
- Hormel Health Labs (www.hormelhealthlabs.com)
- Dysphagia Diet (www.dysphagia-diet.com)
- MultiGen Purées™ (www.multigenpurees.com)

Hydration

There is nothing inherently dehydrating about thickening products. Commercially available thickeners are designed to return essentially all of the fluid to the system, and yet when we put a thick-liquid intervention into place, we may increase our client's risk of dehydration. Why? Some clients simply do not find thick liquids palatable and, in turn, drink less.

The more important issue with pediatric clients, however, is satiety. Thick liquids are more filling, which causes babies and children to drink less. Thick liquids also take longer to digest, so clients stay full longer and reduce their overall intake as a result (Cichero, 2013). Access to liquids is sometimes an issue as well: Given that thickened liquids require preparation, measuring, and mixing, we tend to offer them less frequently than we do regular, unthickened liquids to children without dysphagia. It is important, then, to assist families with developing a plan to maintain hydration whenever you recommend a thick-liquid intervention.

Strategies to Improve Hydration

1. Offer liquids at scheduled times.
2. Set a daily liquid volume goal (with guidance from a dietician or physician).
3. Increase intake of fluid-rich foods (e.g., fruits, vegetables).
4. Offer water throughout the day.
5. Experiment with different liquids, flavors, and thickening products to find fluids most acceptable to your client.
6. Offer smaller (but more frequent) volumes of thickened liquids to reduce satiety.
7. Optimize fluid retention in cooking (e.g., steaming rather than grilling).

Product Issues

Thickening products are notoriously difficult to use. It is challenging to consistently achieve the same consistency when thickening because the products themselves are difficult to mix at times and, more importantly, perform differently with different liquids. The type and temperature of the base liquid, the time post-thickening, and individual product differences can all have an impact on the viscosity of the final product (Payne et al., 2011).

Of particular concern to pediatric therapists is the thickening of breastmilk, which presents additional challenges for a number of reasons. Enzymes in breastmilk break down starches and render starch-based thickeners ineffective. Gum-based thickeners are also not an option, given that xanthan gum has been linked to necrotizing enterocolitis in premature infants, resulting in an FDA warning against its use (Woods et al., 2012). Recently, locust bean gums have been proposed for thickening breastmilk and formula, but no information is available as to their safety in preterm infants.

Baby cereals are also sometimes utilized to thicken expressed breastmilk or formula, but they can be difficult for infants to digest properly. In addition, cereals often separate from liquids over time, and care must be taken to frequently remix the liquid throughout the feeding or to thicken in small batches only. Finally, breastmilk is inherently variable, and it can be difficult to provide guidance to families as to how much thickener to use. The IDDSI guidelines have proposed viscosity testing via flow testing and spoon drip testing to ensure appropriate thickness levels (see https://iddsi.org/ for guidance).

Tips for Using Thickeners

- Read and follow the directions carefully. Many products have different instructions for different base liquids.
- Do not serve liquids thickened with non-cereal products immediately. These products take time to reach their "set" point and, in some cases, continue to thicken for several minutes.
- Stir or vigorously shake the liquid to ensure the thickening agent is well dissolved and the liquid thickens evenly. Consider a whisk or shaker bottle, particularly with gum-type thickeners.

Cost

The cost of thickening varies with the product you are using and the degree of thickness you need to achieve. Insurance plans often do not cover this cost, so it must be assumed by the family, which can create a hardship and may limit their ability to adhere to recommendations in some situations.

Cost of Thickened Liquids

The cost of thickened liquids varies as a function of the product and the viscosity required:

- Starch thickeners: Approximately $0.30/serving
- Gum/gel thickeners: Approximately $0.60/serving
- Pre-thickened beverages: Approximately $1.25/serving

Water: Friend or Foe?

Water, water, everywhere, as the saying goes. Indeed, our bodies are made up largely of water. In babies, almost 80 percent of their weight is water. That gradually drops over the first year of life to about 65 percent, and it continues to drop slowly into adulthood, when approximately 55 to 60 percent of our body weight is water—less for women than men, as we all carry a great deal of water in our muscles and men typically have more muscle.

Our brains and heart are over 70 precent water, and our lungs are over 80 percent water. Water helps us regulate body temperature; gets nutrients where they need to go; gets rid of waste products efficiently; cushions our joints, brain, and spinal cord; forms saliva to lubricate our mouths and throats; and generally keeps our cells and organs doing all the things they need to do. Clearly, we need water! But what about aspiration risk? If our clients are going to aspirate anything, it is likely to be the thinnest of the thin liquids, right?

A great deal of research exists to support the use of free water protocols in adult clients with dysphagia (e.g., Carlaw et al., 2012; Frey & Ramsberger, 2011; Gillman et al., 2017; Karagiannis et al., 2011; Karagiannis & Karagiannis, 2014; Kennedi et al., 2019; Murray et al., 2016; Pooyania et al., 2015). Unrestricted water, in the context of an effective oral hygiene program, does not appear to pose a risk to the lungs of adult clients and, in fact, may decrease dehydration risk and improve quality of life. Unfortunately, in pediatric clients, there is no evidence to support either the use of a water protocol or the restriction of water in clients who are known to aspirate (Weir et al., 2005, 2012). Anecdotally, we know some clinicians use water protocols with pediatric clients, particularly older children whose lungs are presumed to be more adult-like in function, but research in this area is scant.

How do water protocols work? These protocols, which were originally developed for clients with dysphagia at Frazer Rehabilitation Hospital (Panther, 2005), indicate that clients should receive thickened liquids during meals and medication administration times to reduce the risk of choking or aspirating foods or medications. Outside of those times, though, clients are encouraged to drink water—un-thickened water—to improve hydration. Clinicians may put strategies in place to slow the flow or reduce the bolus size, but water is generally unrestricted. A critical aspect of these protocols is regular oral hygiene to reduce the risk of aspiration of oral pathogens.

An advantage of water protocols for pediatric clients is that it affords them an opportunity to practice with thin liquids. Many of our clients have been using thickened liquids since birth (or soon after). They have little to no experience with thin liquids. Water protocols can provide them with opportunities to practice with high-flow, fast-moving thin liquids in a way that reduces the risk of lung infections. As with adult clients, we can choose to use spoon-feeding or slow-flow cups in order to reduce the sip size or to control the flow rate. However, given the lack of research with pediatric clients, it is best to implement water protocols in collaboration with the child's pediatrician or pulmonologist.

ORAL HYGIENE

Good general health depends, in part (some would say in large part), on good oral and dental health. For example, the CDC reports that children with poor oral health miss more school days and have lower grades than children with good oral health (Griffin et al., 2016). In addition, poor oral health has been linked to a variety of health issues, including lung disease and respiratory infections. Pregnant women with poor oral health are also more likely to give birth prematurely. And, of course, good oral hygiene reduces the risk of pneumonia in clients who aspirate. An oral hygiene plan, then, needs to be part of any intervention plan for pediatric clients with pharyngeal dysphagia.

So what does "good" oral hygiene look like? The following table provides recommendations for infants versus toddlers and older children.

Oral Hygiene Recommendations	
Infants	**Toddlers and Older Children**
• Wipe the gums with a wet cloth or use a soft-bristled infant toothbrush after feedings and before sleep. • Caregivers should engage in regular toothbrushing themselves to prevent transfer of bacteria from mouth to mouth. • Brush the infant's teeth twice daily as soon as teeth erupt. Use a very small amount of toothpaste or simply a wet brush with water.	• Brush the teeth a minimum of twice per day, and increase the frequency if aspiration risk is significant. • Use a soft-bristled toothbrush with a small head. • Consider brushing teeth before ingesting food or liquid if the aspiration risk is high. • Get professional teeth cleaning twice a year.

These recommendations can be difficult to implement in practice with children who have sensory processing issues or oral defensiveness. Try using music, incorporating toothbrushes into play activities, and gradually building intraoral acceptance of the brush. For children who are hyposensitive or under-responsive, you can try the following strategies:

- Try tapping, stroking, or vibrating to "alert" the sensory system before oral care. Ideally, provide stimulation to the cheeks and lips, but if the child demonstrates resistance, begin with the hands, arms, or shoulders and slowly move to the face and lips.
- Incorporate physical activity before oral care activities.
- Choose a strongly flavored toothpaste.
- Try a vibrating electric toothbrush.

For children who are hypersensitive or over-responsive, try these strategies to build participation:

- Incorporate calming activities (e.g., deep breathing, squeezes or deep pressure touch to the hands, arms, or face) prior to oral care.
- Choose a low-foam or a mildly flavored toothpaste, or avoid toothpaste altogether.
- Choose a toothbrush with a small head.

Build participation in oral hygiene activities the same way you build participation in eating activities: slowly, over time, and while building on positive experiences.

COMPENSATORY STRATEGIES

Dietary modifications are a large part of pharyngeal dysphagia management in children, but they should not be the *only* thing we do. Compensations involving bolus flow and sensory properties can also be helpful in improving swallow function. As with any exercise or strategy, we always want to be targeted in our approach. Choose your compensation based on the underlying impairment or impairments. So what do we know about what works?

Slow the Flow

We don't have too many one-size-fits-all strategies when it comes to pediatric swallowing disorders, but if we did have one go-to strategy, it would probably be "slow down!" Slowing the liquid flow or the overall pace of intake can compensate for impairments in breathing-swallow coordination, impaired bolus propulsion, delays in airway closure, delays in swallow response initiation, and impairments in pharyngeal transit. We can choose a nipple or cup that allows for a slower flow or impose breaks while the child is eating or drinking.

Reduce Bolus Size

Like a slower flow, smaller bolus sizes can also have a positive impact on pharyngeal swallow function. We can use smaller bites and sips to compensate for impairments in breathing-swallow coordination, impaired bolus control and propulsion, incomplete or delayed airway closure, delays in swallow response initiation, or pharyngeal transit.

Incorporate Sensory Changes

There is a great deal of evidence in adult clients supporting the use of sensory interventions to improve swallow safety. In particular, research shows that manipulating the sensory properties of the bolus can change various aspects of the swallow response. Changing the taste, temperature, and chemesthetic properties of the bolus have been demonstrated to improve lingual-palatal contact and bolus propulsion, the timing of the swallow response, and the timing of airway closure.

Although there is less research in pediatric populations, the evidence we do have lines up with what we know about adult populations. In particular, cold boluses can improve swallow response in infants (Ferrara et al., 2018), and carbonation has been demonstrated to decrease pharyngeal residue and reduce aspiration in children with neurological impairment (Lundine et al., 2015). Therefore, trials of cold foods and liquids, carbonated beverages, and high-flavor foods have the potential to improve swallow safety in pediatric clients by increasing sensory input into the swallow system.

Promote Self-Feeding

Another way to increase sensory input during feeding tasks is to promote self-feeding whenever and to whatever extent possible. Self-feeding alerts the sensory system and increases the child's ability to anticipate and prepare for the food or liquid, which promotes better oral bolus control and swallow safety. In children for whom self-feeding is not possible, consider guided hand-over-hand feeding as a way to provide that sensory input and cueing.

SKILLS TRAINING

What about practice? Does practice make perfect when it comes to swallowing? It looks like that may indeed be the case.

Effortful Swallow

There is evidence in adult patients with dysphagia that effortful swallow can improve overall swallow function (Bahia & Lowell, 2020). Swallowing "hard," or with effort, is in many ways the quintessential exercise. It is easy to understand and accomplish, can be done with any bolus type, requires no equipment, and has perfect specificity in that it encompasses each discrete aspect of the swallow and adds effort. What we know from research with adults is that effortful swallow has the potential to improve lingual-palatal contact and subsequent bolus propulsion, facilitate pharyngeal transit, improve airway closure and protection, and improve hyolaryngeal excursion.

Bolus Hold

We again turn to the adult literature for guidance on bolus holding, which tells us that increasing oral bolus control can improve pharyngeal swallow safety (Nagy et al., 2013). Instructing clients to "hold" the food or liquid in their mouths for two to three seconds before swallowing can improve oral bolus containment and reduce pre-swallow entry to the pharynx, and it can also improve airway protection and airway closure. Use a verbal prompt like "one, two three, swallow" or "hold, hold, go."

These strategies, of course, require volitional control and active participation on the part of our clients. You're probably thinking, *My client is too young to do this* or *My client doesn't have the cognitive ability to follow these directions.* For these clients, skill building is still possible, but clearly, we need an alternative: gradual thinning.

Gradual Thinning

Recently, researchers working with children with pharyngeal dysphagia have reported success with gradually thinning thick liquids until they become thin in viscosity (Wolter et al., 2018). By simply having children consume progressively thinner liquids, they can practice a variety of skills, including bolus control, swallow initiation, and airway protection and airway closure. As children improve and build proficiency, the liquid can be slowly and progressively thinned to continue providing skills training in a controlled manner.

Oral Stimulation

Oral play and stimulation can increase saliva production and therefore increase saliva swallows. Vibration, chewing practice, and taste stimulation can all be used to increase the frequency of swallowing and provide practice. Foods that the feeder can maintain control of, like a lollipop, are ideal for this. The child is able to taste the food without needing to manipulate it or actually swallow it, which increases saliva production and saliva swallows.

Dry Utensil Practice

Training with utensils without food or liquid can provide safe opportunities for children to practice swallowing. An empty cup or a dry spoon can be used to increase the child's familiarity and comfort with the utensil as well as to promote lip closure and tongue movement. As the child progresses, small boluses (e.g., dipping the spoon into a flavored liquid) can be added and steadily increased to build bolus management skills and swallow safety.

UTENSIL CHOICE

The choice of utensil is an important tool in the management of pharyngeal dysphagia and aspiration risk. For example, a cup that slows the flow of the liquid, such as a covered cup, can assist in improving bolus control and airway protection. An alternative to a covered cup is a cut-out cup that allows the feeder to squeeze the edges of the cup together to slow the flow.

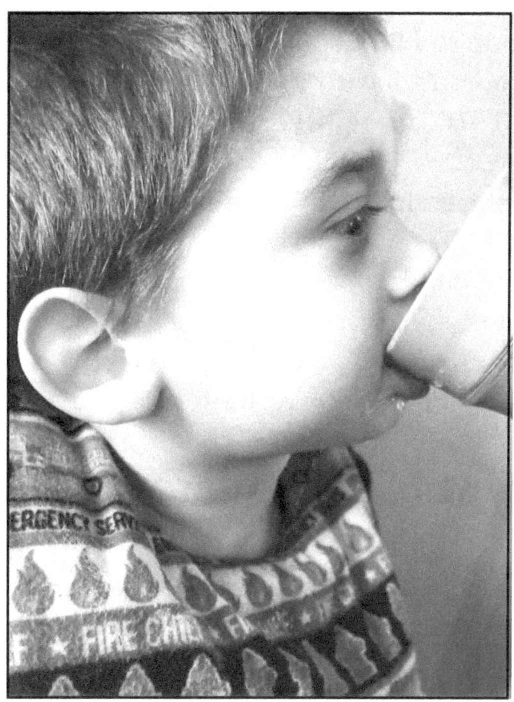

Straw use should be evaluated on a case-by-case basis and confirmed for safety via instrumental assessment whenever possible. For some children, straws have the potential to improve pharyngeal swallow safety as they allow the child to use a natural chin-down head position, which provides added protection to the airway. A straw with a smaller diameter can also help reduce bolus flow and sip size. Straw drinking can be particularly helpful when paired with a straw block to reduce the amount of straw that is actually in the mouth—in other words, to ensure that bolus delivery is near the front of the mouth rather than the back.

For some children, though, there is a concern about straws related to bolus placement. In particular, straw drinking has the potential to deliver the bolus farther back in the mouth and may increase the likelihood of pre-swallow spill to the pharynx. In fact, straw drinking with healthy subjects has been demonstrated to increase early entry to the pharynx and to increase pharyngeal "dwell time"—the length of time the liquid sits in the pharynx before the swallow response triggers (Daniels & Foundas, 2001). In those of us with healthy swallows, this is not a problem, but in a child who already has some delay or inefficiency in their swallow response, straw drinking may increase their risk.

Feeding therapists often use cups or bottles with straws with one-way valves to teach straw drinking. These valves keep the liquid near the top of the straw so the child doesn't have to draw liquid through the length of the straw for every sip. This can be helpful for children with oral motor issues. These cups also allow the feeder to squeeze small amounts of liquid into the child's mouth while the child is still learning to draw liquid into their mouth. However, care must be taken when working with children with pharyngeal dysphagia. The feeder should practice with the cup or bottle prior to placing it in the child's mouth. We want to avoid overfilling the child's mouth or squeezing liquid into the child's mouth too quickly, as this could result in a loss of bolus control and potential aspiration or choking.

GASTROESOPHAGEAL REFLUX DISEASE AND PHARYNGEAL SWALLOWING

The complications associated with GERD are varied and can impact the upper airway in the form of voice changes, ear infections, and throat pain. GERD can also exacerbate pharyngeal dysphagia. Regular, or even intermittent, acid exposure to the larynx and pharynx can result in swelling and mucosal damage than can cause or worsen aspiration risk. Therefore, strategies that help bring the GERD under better control can also improve pharyngeal swallow safety (Suskind et al., 2006). See chapter 3 for a full discussion of GERD management strategies.

POSITIONING

In general, a more upright position is recommended to improve bolus control and airway protection. Avoid positioning the child with their head extended, as this may decrease oral control and increase choking risk. Some children will need supports to maintain a comfortable, stable position throughout the feeding. You can find a full discussion of positioning strategies and suggestions in chapter 5.

NON-ORAL FEEDING

In very severe cases of pharyngeal dysphagia, you may determine that oral feeding is unsafe despite dietary modifications or compensatory strategies. In those cases, non-oral feeding may be recommended. However, even children who are non-oral feeders will continue to benefit from oral stimulation and, in some cases, oral feeding in small amounts. If the goal is to help the child wean from the feeding tube and transition to oral feeding, practice will be necessary. Chapter 7 provides a more detailed discussion regarding the delivery of nutrition via a feeding tube and also presents strategies for weaning.

5

Slurp, Chew, and Bite: Improving Oral Motor Function

MUSCLES AND MOVEMENT

Let's talk about muscles: What do we know? How do they work? Why do they work? As we begin, let's define some important terms relevant to muscle movements and exercise:

Speed	• Maximal velocity
Force	• Ability to transfer energy (i.e., push or pull) • Changes motion, speed, direction
Strength	• The force-generating capacity of a muscle
Power	• Ability to exert force quickly • Strength + speed
Endurance	• Ability to continually produce force over a long period of time (what defines "long" varies with the activity) • Stamina

We know that our bodies are made up of muscles and that those muscles are made up of fibers. The muscle fibers require innervation, and that innervation is achieved via *motor neurons*. A muscle fiber is innervated by a single motor neuron, but a single motor neuron can be responsible for many fibers. The motor neuron is made up of three components: the cell body, the dendrites, and the axon. The dendrites receive signals from other neurons while the axon transmits information to and from the muscle fibers. When triggered by a stimulus, electrical activity travels from the cell body down the axon to the muscle fibers, which is referred to as an *action potential* or *nerve impulse*.

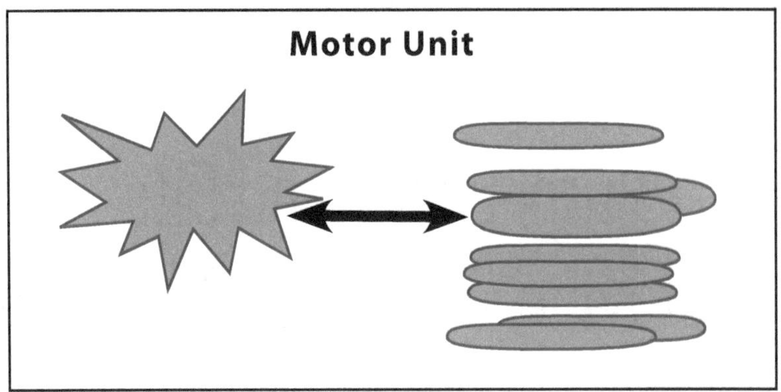

A motor neuron and the fibers for which it is responsible make up a *motor unit*. There are different numbers and types of motor units in our muscles, depending on the location, size, and purpose of the muscle. Motor units function as a whole and are "recruited" or called into play for specific movements and movement patterns throughout motor planning systems. Recruitment becomes more efficient with repetition. In other words, the more you practice a movement, the more efficient your recruitment becomes—and the more efficient your recruitment becomes, the more efficient your movement becomes.

There are three agreed-upon categories of motor units: Type I, Type IIa, and Type IIb. Each has a different role to play when it comes to muscle movements. Motor units are categorized according to their speed or "twitch." Those that are classified as "slow twitch" are slower to result in muscle tension, while those that are "fast twitch" create muscle tension more quickly. Motor units are also described according to their fatigue resistance. Some motor units are more efficient at protein metabolism and are therefore less susceptible to fatigue. This makes them more suitable for tasks that require more prolonged activity.

Categories of Motor Units		
Type I	**Type IIa**	**Type IIb**
• Slow twitch • Slow to fatigue • Are the first to be recruited and remain recruited throughout the task • Best for activities requiring endurance • Less suited for high-force activities	• Fast twitch • Intermediate response to fatigue • Recruited after Type I motor units but before Type IIb	• Fast twitch • Quick to fatigue • Are the last to be recruited and the first to fatigue • High potential for force generation

All muscles contain all three motor unit types in different proportions, depending on the muscle's function. For example, muscles that are responsible for faster movements would contain more Type IIa and Type IIb motor units. In general, head and neck muscles contain more Type II motor units than Type I, but they also have some additional unique characteristics. Head and neck muscles are certainly smaller than skeletal muscles and contain fibers that are hybrids of Type I and Type II units. This may explain why the head and neck muscles are significantly resistant against fatigue. (And it explains why we can talk all day without tiring out our tongues!)

What Happens When We Move Our Muscles?

In order to move our muscles, we go through the following five steps:

1. A message regarding our intent to move is sent from the central nervous system to the muscles via nerve impulses, or action potentials.
2. That impulse continues and is transmitted across the neuromuscular junction (via release of acetylcholine, which is an important neurotransmitter).
3. The impulse transmission continues into the muscle.
4. This triggers a chemical reaction within the muscle fibers.
5. The fibers innervated by that motor neuron then contract as a unit and the muscle moves.

Simple, right? But what do we do for our clients who can't do that efficiently? We help them exercise those muscles. We generally think of exercise as a structured plan for repetitive movement that can improve muscle functions (as well as our overall health). You might be wondering if exercise has application to our work with feeding and swallowing impairments in pediatric clients. And if so, you might be wondering which clients are appropriate candidates. Let's talk about what we know.

EXERCISE

What Happens When We Exercise?

The impact of exercise on our muscle fibers depends on the type of exercise being conducted:

- Endurance exercises increase the number of Type I fibers.
- Resistance exercises increase the number of Type II fibers.
- Repeated voluntary movements recruit both (Type I first, then Type II).

In order for exercise to be effective, we need to have some assurance that we are recruiting all of the available motor units. Change in motor function occurs when we push the system to overload. In other words, the exercise has to be hard, and we need to do a lot of it. That means thinking about the *intensity* of the activity. Whatever we choose has to exceed the typical demand we put on the muscles. We also need to consider *exercise frequency*, or the number of training sessions in any given period of time. This includes the number of repetitions we do and the number of times per day we complete those repetitions. Finally, we need assurance that we can incorporate *progression* into our program. Systematic increases in resistance, duration, and number of repetitions ensure that we are continually pushing the system to overload and maximizing our potential to change muscle function.

How Do We Choose a Target?

Think about your personal experiences with exercise. You've learned that if you want to increase your strength, the best way to do so is with resistance training. And you know that if you want to improve your endurance, the best way to do that is to complete more repetitions.

Well, what is it that your client needs? Are you trying to build strength? Then your activity needs to include resistance. Are you trying to improve endurance? Then you need to focus on increasing the number of repetitions your client can complete. Or are you trying to train (or re-train) a specific sequence of movements, like chewing or bolus manipulation? If that's the case, then that specific sequence *is* your exercise. Turns out, if we want our clients to get better at chewing, they need to chew. If we want them to get better at swallowing liquids, they need to swallow liquids. If we want them to improve their ability to manipulate food in their mouth, then that's exactly what we need to practice. We make it an exercise by doing a lot of it (frequency) and by making it harder to do (intensity), but the task has to contain the basic components of the target motor task.

That's because *specificity* is an important principle of exercise physiology. In other words: Exercise doesn't generalize. That means we need to target the muscles exhibiting the weakness as well as the specific movement sequence that is deficient. Generalized tongue movement and oral play is fun, but it won't improve your client's ability to move food onto their teeth for chewing. Repeating the "t" sound requires tongue tip elevation, but it won't help with the elevation required to start a swallow. In fact, motor control for speech and non-speech mechanisms have completely different neural controls.

Principles of Neuroplasticity

The principles of neuroplasticity—in other words, the things that get our brain to change—are similar to the principles of exercise physiology:

- **Reversibility:** Use it or lose it.
- **Repetition:** Use it and improve it.
- **Specificity:** Practice what you want to improve.
- **Variety:** Multiple planes facilitate recruitment of motor units.
- **Intensity:** Exercise has to be hard to do.

Our goal, of course, is to improve function. However, when it comes to feeding and swallowing exercises, we will first see behavioral plasticity before we see muscular and neural plasticity. The behavior changes, the task becomes easier, and compensations are utilized. With repetition of the activity, we then expect to see muscular plasticity. The muscle changes, becomes stronger, and has more endurance. Structurally, we see capillaries increase and provide more oxygenation, and we see muscle fiber diameter increase, which results in improved function.

With maintenance of the muscular plasticity, we then see neural plasticity or brain change. What happens when brains change? Protein synthesis in the brain becomes more efficient, new synapses are generated, and the cortical map reorganizes. In other words, brain cells take on new functions. In order for neuroplastic changes to occur, though, habilitation (or rehabilitation) must be done in the context of a healthy cortex. The potential for plasticity is different at different developmental timepoints, but fortunately for those of us who work with children, younger brains are generally more amenable to change.

Who Is a Good Candidate for Exercise?

When we are considering an exercise (or exercises) for a particular client, we first have to ask ourselves if the client is an appropriate candidate for an exercise intervention:

- Clients with *weakness or low endurance* are generally good candidates, as these are deficits that exercise can target. However, we must ask ourselves about the etiology of the weakness. Is this a client who is likely to improve? Or are we expecting continual decline given the progressive nature of the disorder?

- Clients who demonstrate the potential to complete activities with *high frequency and intensity* are also good candidates. This often eliminates clients with low cognition who can't follow directions or clients whose deficits are so severe that they cannot produce even an approximation of the movement.

What Makes a Good Exercise?

When determining what constitutes a good exercise, ask yourself the following questions:

- Can this activity be done with high frequency? Can my particular client achieve that?
- Is this activity hard to do? (In other words, can it be done with intensity?)
- Can I progress this and make it continually more difficult to ensure I am recruiting all of the available motor units?
- Does it have specificity? How is it related to the specific skill I am interested in training (or re-training)?

SKILLS TRAINING: A CHANGE IN FOCUS

In the rehabilitation research, the focus has recently changed from exercise to skills training. The goal of skills training is the acquisition (or re-acquisition) of a specific skill or set of skills. The task is continually refined and fine-tuned until the client has met the goal and acquired the target skill. Biofeedback is often incorporated to ensure that task performance is accurate and to improve retention of the motor pattern.

Skills training incorporates the principles of motor learning:

- **Attention and motivation:** You can't learn what you're not paying attention to.
- **Structured practice:** Regular performance of the task allows us to continually refine our movements.
- **Specificity:** Practice what you want to improve.
- **Repetition at high intensity:** Activities have to be harder to do than the actual functional activity.

- **Increasing challenge for refinement of task:** Shape the task to get closer and closer to the goal movement or movements.
- **Feedback:** In order to learn to do it right, you have to *know* when you're doing it right.

Sounds similar to exercise physiology, right? But the focus is on motor planning rather than strengthening. *Cortical* learning is the goal.

PUTTING PRINCIPLES INTO PRACTICE

How do we operationalize all of these principles? What do we actually do as we sit across from our clients? First, we want to think about our method of instruction. We want to balance instructions and prompting with room for error. After all, we learn as much from our mistakes as we do from our successes (maybe more, in fact). There is also some evidence to suggest that changing up the sequence in which you practice the activities can facilitate learning. Performing tasks in the exact same way and in the exact same order results in rigidity in learning. By mixing up the practice tasks, we can build skills that last.

We also want to think about our method of exercise. Feeding therapists have historically found themselves conflicted about exercise. One theory holds that remediation is best accomplished at the task level (e.g., practice chewing to improve chewing; practice swallowing to improve swallowing), which gets back to the specificity principle. On the other hand, we know that the underlying impairment in neuromuscular function contributes to the disability and should be addressed. Breaking down complex skills into manageable chunks and training those underlying skills should result in improvement as a whole, right? So which is it? The answer may lie in the whole-part-whole method. Practice the functional task, then practice individual components, then practice the task again.

Activities to Improve Jaw Function

When putting the principles of exercise into practice, it is helpful to start by thinking about exactly what we need our client to be able to do and what is not working as it should. For example, what do we need the jaw to do? The jaw is important for biting and chewing, and it provides stability so the lips and tongue can function optimally. The following table describes several activities to improve jaw function, depending on your specific goal area.

Goal Area	Activity	Tool(s)	Verbal Instructions	Strategies for Progression
Lateral bite	Place an item on the side of the mouth on the back teeth. Instruct your client to bite down and hold for several seconds. Relax. Move to the other side and repeat. Continue for several repetitions, alternating sides.	• Chewy tubing • High-texture food (e.g., carrot, jerky)	• "Bite and hold." • "Use your teeth and don't let go."	• Increase the number of trials. • Increase the duration of the bite. • Choose a thicker, more fibrous item.
Lateral bite	Place item on the side of the mouth on the back teeth. Instruct your client to bite down *on both pieces simultaneously*, hold for several seconds, and relax. Repeat for several trials.	• Chewy tubing • High-texture food (e.g., carrot, jerky)	• "Bite and hold." • "Use your teeth and don't let go."	• Increase the number of trials. • Increase the duration of the bite. • Choose a thicker, more fibrous item.
Lateral bite	Place an item on the side of the mouth on the back teeth. Instruct your client to bite down and hold for several seconds while you tug on the tubing to *provide resistance*. Relax. Move to the other side and repeat. Continue for several repetitions, alternating sides.	• Chewy tubing • High-texture food (e.g., carrot, jerky)	• "Bite and hold." • "Use your teeth and don't let go." • "Don't let me have it!"	• Increase the number of trials. • Increase the duration of the bite. • Choose a thicker, more fibrous item. • Increase the amount of resistance you provide.

Goal Area	**Activity**	**Tool(s)**	**Verbal Instructions**	**Strategies for Progression**
Lateral bite	Place two pieces of chewy tubing or food on the side of the mouth on the back teeth. Instruct your client to bite down on *both pieces simultaneously* and to hold for several seconds while you tug on the food or tubing to *provide resistance*. Relax, and repeat for several trials.	• Chewy tubing • High-texture food (e.g., carrot, jerky)	• "Bite and hold." • "Use your teeth and don't let go." • "Don't let me have it!"	• Increase the number of trials. • Increase the duration of the bite. • Choose a thicker, more fibrous item. • Increase the amount of resistance you provide.
Anterior (front) bite	As lateral bite strength increases, continue with the above activities, alternating sides and gradually *moving closer to the front of the mouth.*	• Chewy tubing • High-texture food (e.g., carrot, jerky)	• "Bite and hold." • "Use your teeth and don't let go." • "Don't let me have it!"	• Increase the number of trials. • Increase the duration of the bite. • Choose a thicker, more fibrous item. • Increase the amount of resistance you provide.
Anterior (front) bite	Place foods at the front of the mouth and instruct your client to "take a bite."	Foods of various thicknesses or textures	• "Bite and hold." • "Use your teeth and don't let go." • "Don't let me have it!"	• Increase the texture. • Increase the thickness. • Increase the number of repetitions.

Goal Area	Activity	Tool(s)	Verbal Instructions	Strategies for Progression
Jaw stability	Instruct your client to open their mouth incrementally, holding in place at each increment until fully open. Then have them close incrementally, holding in place at each increment until fully closed. Relax and repeat.	Consider a puppet to demonstrate partial opening and closing. Best done in front of a mirror.	• "Open a little bit." • "Hold, hold, hold." • "Open all the way." • "Hold, hold, hold." • "Close partway." • "Hold, hold, hold." • "Close all the way and relax."	• Increase the number of repetitions. • Increase the duration of the hold time. • Increase the number of opening or closing increments.
Jaw stability	Instruct your client to move their tongue from side to side inside the mouth *without moving the jaw*. Place your hands on their jaw to reduce movement if necessary.	Best done in front of a mirror	• "Touch your tongue inside your cheek here." • "Now touch your other cheek." • "Wag back and forth." • "Move just your tongue."	• Increase the number of repetitions. • Increase the speed of tongue movement. • Reduce external assistance.

Goal Area	Activity	Tool(s)	Verbal Instructions	Strategies for Progression
Chewing	Place an item in the mouth along the right side. Instruct your client to chew on the item for several repetitions. Move the item to the other side of the mouth, and instruct your client to chew on this side for several repetitions. Continue for several repetitions, alternating sides.	• Chewy tubing • Consider dipping in puree or juice for flavor	• "Use your tongue to scoop this up." • "Move it over to your cheek." • "Chew, chew, chew." • "Don't stop until you've moved it over here." • Consider tapping on the external cheek to provide a target.	• Increase the number of repetitions. • Increase the weight of the item. • Incorporate tongue lateralization activities simultaneously.
Chewing	Place foods laterally, as far back on the molars as you can. Encourage your client to chew. Repeat on the opposite side.	Begin with dissolvable boluses (e.g., puffs, freeze-dried fruit, small pieces of cracker), and advance to foods of higher texture	• "Chew, chew, chew."	• Increase the number of repetitions. • Increase the fibrousness and texture of foods presented. • Increase the size of the bolus presented.

Activities to Improve Tongue Function

What are the functions of the tongue? In infants, the primary function of the tongue is sucking, whereas in children, the focus is on bolus lateralization and manipulation and bolus propulsion. The following table provides several activities that can help you improve functioning in each of these areas.

Goal Area	Activity	Tool(s)	Verbal Instructions	Strategies for Progression
Sucking*	Non-nutritive sucking	Pacifier	N/A	N/A
Bolus lateralization/ manipulation	Place an item in the middle of the mouth. Instruct your client to move the item to the right side of the mouth *using only the tongue*. Relax and repeat, moving the item to the other side. Continue for several repetitions.	Pacifier	• "Use your tongue to scoop this up." • "Move it over to your cheek." • Consider tapping on the external cheek to provide a target.	• Increase the number of repetitions. • Increase the weight of the item. • Add resistance by pushing back against the tongue movement.
Bolus lateralization/ manipulation	Place an item in the mouth along the right side. Instruct your client to move the item across midline to the other side of the mouth *using only the tongue*. Encourage smooth movement without a midline stop when possible. Continue for several repetitions.	Pacifier	• "Use your tongue to scoop this up." • "Move it over to your cheek." • Consider tapping on the external cheek to provide a target. • "Don't stop until you've moved it over here."	• Increase the number of repetitions. • Increase the weight of the item. • Add resistance by pushing back against the tongue movement. • Incorporate chewing activities simultaneously.
Bolus propulsion	Instruct your client to swallow with effort.	Any bolus determined to be safe for your client to swallow	• "Hold in your mouth for a second…now swallow hard!"	• Increase the number of repetitions. • Increase the size of the bolus.
Bolus propulsion	Ask the client to press their tongue against the roof of their mouth.	Small solid boluses	• "Push hard against the top of your mouth."	• Increase the number of repetitions.
Bolus management/ lip clearance	Place a small amount of puree on the client's lips in various locations. Ask the client to use their tongue to clear/clean the puree.	Any pureed bolus	• "Use your tongue." • "Clean it off."	• Increase the number of repetitions. • Increase the viscosity of the food.

* The evidence for the use of non-nutritive sucking is inconclusive as it relates to tongue strengthening for nutritive sucking. It does, however, appear to improve state regulation and tongue functions.

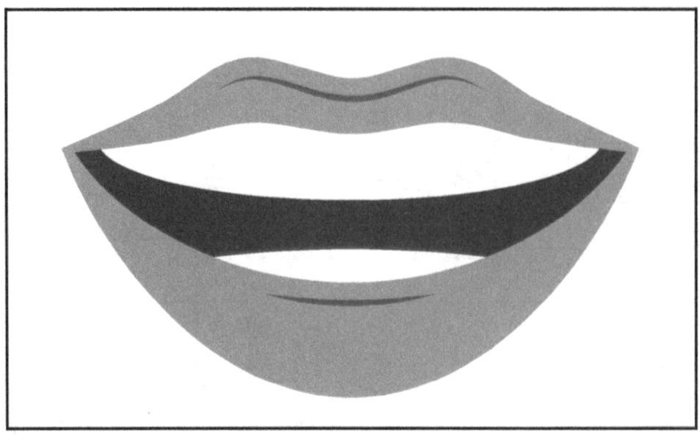

Activities to Improve Lip Function

What do we need our lips for? Mostly for closure. We need our lips to close around a straw, to close on and clear a spoon, and to stay closed while we're eating. The following table provides activities to help your clients achieve goals with regard to spoon clearance and straw sipping.

Goal Area	Activity	Tool(s)	Verbal Instructions	Strategies for Progression
Spoon clearance	Place a spoon with bolus in the client's mouth at midline.	Spoons with bowls of varying depths and boluses of various thicknesses	• "Lips together." • "Use your lips, not your teeth."	• Increase the number of repetitions. • Increase bowl depth. • Increase the viscosity of the bolus.
Straw sips	Place a straw in the client's mouth and encourage closure.	Straws of varying diameters	• "Lips together." • "Use your lips, not your teeth."	• If the client is having difficulty, place the straw slightly off midline and work toward midline as lip function improves. • Increase the number of repetitions. • Decrease the diameter of the straw.

Biofeedback

If we want our clients to perform a given task correctly, they need to *know* when they are doing it correctly. Our verbal prompts and praise are often not enough. It is here that biofeedback can help clients identify their ability to accurately complete a task. The evidence about when to provide feedback is mixed: Some evidence suggests that immediate feedback is best, while some supports the idea of delayed feedback.

All of this research, however, has been completed with adults, so we know far less about motor learning in pediatric clients. What we do know is that a number of variables can impact learning in children, including attention and developmental stage, so we need to tailor whatever feedback we provide to the specific learning needs of our client. Consider using a mirror, as this may be the best way to provide immediate feedback. Videotaping the activity for review later may work better for older children. When available, electromyography (EMG) can also provide feedback for swallowing tasks like effortful swallow.

Exercise Dose

When it comes to feeding and swallowing exercises, clinicians must consider the following questions: What is the appropriate number of repetitions for each activity? How many times a day should the client perform the activities? These are questions related to exercise "dose." Body builders know just how many repetitions of a particular exercise they should do to complete a set, what the rest period between sets should be, and how many sets should be completed in a day. When it comes to head and neck muscles, though, we don't have that kind of information yet. So how do we guide our clients and their parents? How much exercise is appropriate?

If we remember that the goal of exercise is to push the system to overload—to recruit every available motor unit—then the appropriate dose is the number of repetitions that will push this child's system to fatigue. How many trials does it take to push this child to fatigue while performing a particular exercise or activity? That number is the dose for that child.

FACILITATING TRANSITIONS TO NEW FOODS AND UTENSILS

Just as important as finding the right activity or exercise is understanding when and how to move on to a more challenging task, food, or utensil. It is helpful to keep the following "typical" developmental sequence in mind, always understanding that there is a great deal of variability when it comes to what is considered "typical":

- Nipple-fed liquid
- Puree via spoon
- Liquids from a cup
- Chewables
- Liquids via straw
- Biteable foods
- Mixed-texture foods
- Foods that require extended chewing

In general, we want to move the child from one texture to the next and from one utensil to the next. For the most part, we want to remain within the developmental sequence, but we may make exceptions in certain cases. For example, toddlers who are G-tube dependent for several years may never really learn to suck or suckle but will transition directly to purees or soft solid foods and liquids from a cup. Similarly, children who struggle with a cup because of their oral motor deficits may actually perform better with a straw, even though it is a later developing skill.

Typically, we make one transition at a time. If you are trying a new food, try it with a familiar utensil. If you are trying a new utensil, do it with a food or liquid that the child has experience with. And in all cases, make sure the child is ready to make that transition. Readiness requires physiological stability, environmental preparedness, and an ability and desire to meet the task requirements.

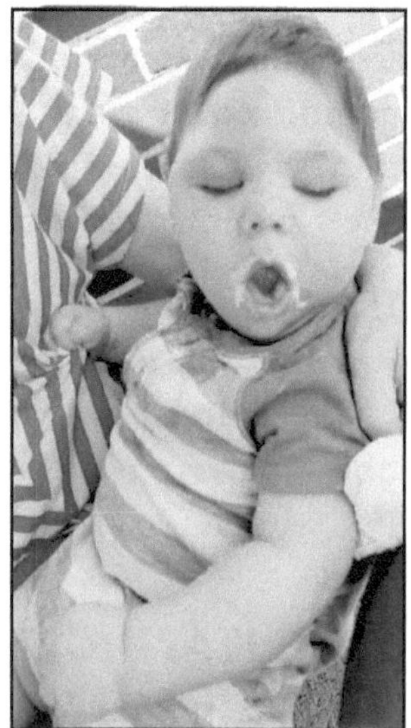

Readiness for Transitions

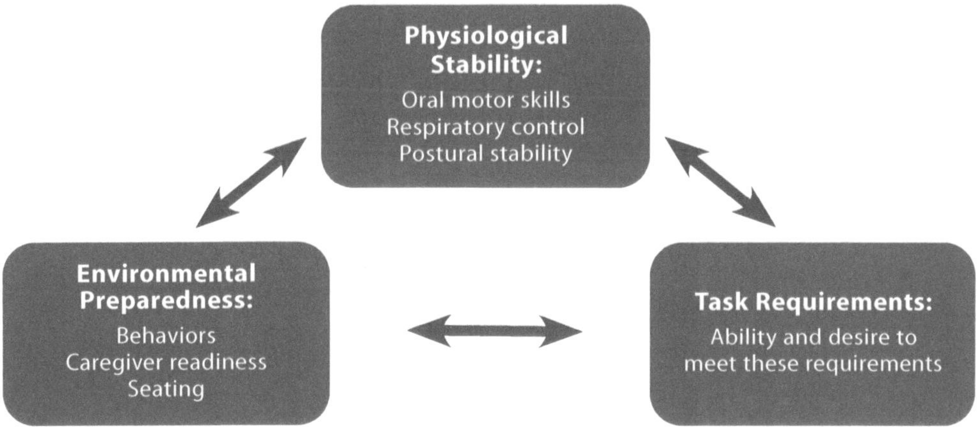

Physiological Stability:
Oral motor skills
Respiratory control
Postural stability

Environmental Preparedness:
Behaviors
Caregiver readiness
Seating

Task Requirements:
Ability and desire to meet these requirements

You may have a client, for example, who appears ready for more textured foods. She has the oral motor skills needed to meet the task requirements. However, her preschool classroom only has benches at snack tables that do not provide enough postural stability, and she is not successful. Or perhaps you are treating a client who appears ready for open-cup practice, but his parents are reluctant to provide the practice opportunities because they don't want him to make a mess. Environmental readiness is clearly a critical factor in helping our clients to make successful transitions.

As you work through each transition, it is important to identify the child's readiness signs and to provide strategies to facilitate the transition. The following section provides examples of the readiness signals for various types of transitions, including the transition to nippling, spoon feeding, cup drinking, chewing, straw drinking, and biting.

Transition to Liquids via Nipple

Readiness Signs

- Effective, rhythmic non-nutritive sucking
- Medical stability (maintains stable vital signs during feeding trials)
- Stable respiratory system
- Tolerates normal feeding schedule for non-oral feeds
- Able to maintain calm, awake state
- Rooting (opening mouth for nipple)

How can we facilitate effective sucking in infants? As discussed in chapter 3, slowing the flow is a critical strategy for promoting respiratory stability. Additional strategies that can facilitate a calm, ready state and improve sucking include trials with rhythm, music, and rocking. Finally, positioning is important to a successful transition to nippling. Elevated side-lying can promote respiratory stability and improve pharyngeal swallow function.

Transition to Spoon Feeding

Readiness Signs

- Anterior-posterior tongue mobility for bolus transfer
- Opens mouth in anticipation of bolus and leans in toward spoon
- Attempts to suck off spoon
- Able to close lips around spoon
- Emerging jaw stability

You can facilitate spoon feeding by incorporating spoons into play, particularly in oral play. Practice with a dry spoon by having clients accept the spoon in their mouths and close around the spoon without the demand of a bolus. Presenting the longer lateral edge of the spoon against the lips provides more surface area and improves jaw stability, which in turn improves upper lip function for closure and clearance.

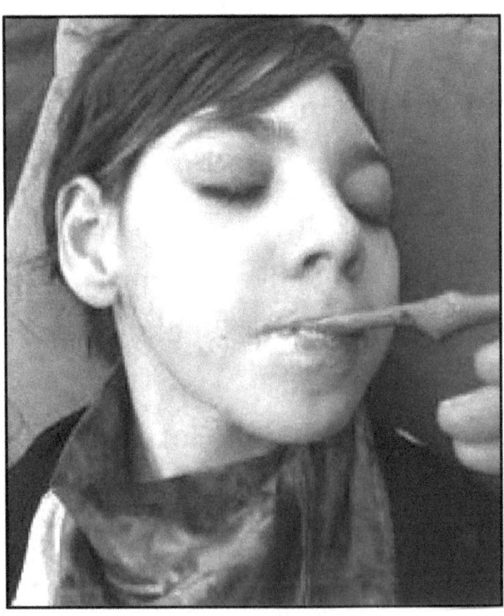

Spoon choice is an additional consideration. Be sure the bowl of the spoon is appropriate for the child's age and individual anatomy. Pay attention to the depth of the bowl in particular. The deeper the bowl, the more upper lip movement is required. For children with oral weakness and inefficiencies, consider a spoon with a shallower bowl or a completely flat spoon. A deeper spoon can increase sensory input but will be more difficult to clear. To increase sensory information for the child without increasing motor demand, choose a spoon that is shallower but has ridges or texture. You can also modify the food itself—choose colder or more highly flavored foods—to increase sensory information in a shallower spoon.

Transition to Cup Drinking

Readiness Signs

- Moves toward cup when offered and closes mouth around cup lip
- Attempts jaw closure on rim of cup
- Emerging jaw stability

Utensil choice is important for cup drinking as well. Consider what you know about your client's oral motor function, specifically their potential for lingual control and jaw stability. If you have concerns about lingual control, you will have to choose a cup that allows you to control and slow the flow. Choose a covered cup or a small open cup that will give the feeder control over the flow rate. If jaw stability is not complete, the child will have to stabilize *against* the cup in order to achieve controlled lip and tongue movements. A more rigid cup, then, will be more appropriate. A cup with a recessed lid provides more surface area and can also improve jaw stability and support. Of course, you may have reductions in both jaw stability and lingual mobility and will have to choose a rigid or recessed cup lid with flow control.

When practicing cup sips, try to leave the cup in place whenever possible. Every time you remove the cup and replace it in position, the child has to reestablish jaw stability and positioning. It is not always possible to leave the cup in place, but when this can be achieved, it can improve jaw function and subsequently lingual and labial functions. An additional consideration is the liquid choice. As you transition to faster-flow cups, it can be helpful to start with a naturally thicker liquid, such as milk rather than water or a yogurt drink rather than juice.

Transition to Chewing

Readiness Signs

- Emerging lateral tongue movements
- Vertical jaw movements
- Interest in and acceptance of texture

Chewing skills can be facilitated in two ways: via food placement and food choice. We can place foods laterally, on the back molars if possible, to encourage vertical jaw movement. Alternate sides when placing food in the child's mouth to ensure adequate bilateral practice and to promote rotary jaw movements. Lateral food placement will also stimulate tongue lateralization for better overall bolus management.

When it comes to food choice, foods that are dissolvable are good selections for initial trials because they will melt into puree form if the child is not able to control the bolus adequately. Cohesive foods also make good choices, as they will stay together and therefore require less lingual manipulation. As trials progress, choose foods of gradually increasing texture.

Examples of Dissolvable Foods

- Gerber® Puffs
- Pirate's Booty®
- Small pieces of cracker
- EAT Bars
- Freeze-dried fruits
- Savorease crackers

Transition to Straw Drinking

Readiness Signs

- Managing liquids from a cup
- Able to achieve or approximate labial closure
- Emerging jaw stability

There are two aspects of straw drinking to consider: labial closure and ability to draw through the straw. We can improve labial closure around the straw by adjusting the diameter of the straw. Wider straws are good starting places because they are easier to close around. In addition, you can experiment with straw placement by placing the straw off midline, which can facilitate improved closure.

To facilitate the child's ability to draw through the straw, reduce the length of the straw. One-way valves are available that only allow liquid to flow up the straw. The liquid will not flow back down the straw when the child removes their lips or stops sucking. This allows the child to draw from nearer to the top of the straw.

Transition to Biting

Readiness Signs

- Successfully managing chewables
- Emerging jaw stability
- Beginning to exhibit graded jaw movements

Like chewing, biting can be facilitated via food choices and food placement. Choose foods of steadily increasing texture and bolus size to facilitate management of more highly textured, fibrous foods. As the child transitions from chewing to biting trials, continue to place food in their mouth laterally, alternate sides, and gradually move forward in the mouth. Bite strength typically develops laterally, then anteriorly, so begin with lateral bite and slowly move forward, transitioning to anterior bite.

COMPENSATION: WHEN EXERCISE ISN'T THE ANSWER

Exercise and skills training are not quick fixes, and as we've established, not every child will be an appropriate candidate given their cognitive capacity, attentional span, or ability to follow directions (or lack thereof). Resist the temptation to create a long list of strategies that will be difficult for parents and caregivers to complete. Be targeted in your strategy choice, and ask yourself: What is the underlying deficit? What is it I want to compensate for? You can use the following table as guide when making this determination.

Underlying Deficit	Compensatory Strategies
Difficulty with oral bolus propulsion	• Change bolus type: Choose purees and dissolvable solids, or consider naturally thicker liquids. • Change bolus size: Reduce size. • Change bolus placement: Consider more posterior placement on the tongue. Providing downward pressure on the tongue with a spoon can reduce anterior tongue movement and facilitate propulsion. • Change utensil: Consider a spoon with a deeper bowl or textured bottom to facilitate a more retracted tongue position. Choose a cup that allows for a slower flow.
Limited bolus lateralization	• Change bolus type: Choose purees or dissolvable solids. • Change bolus size: Reduce size. • Change bolus placement: Place the bolus on the client's teeth to stimulate tongue lateralization and to avoid mashing against palate.
Limited chew	• Change bolus type: Choose soft or dissolvable solids, and consider crunchy foods to provide auditory feedback. • Change bolus size: Reduce size. • Change bolus placement: Place the bolus laterally to facilitate vertical jaw movement, and alternate sides.
Reduced bite	• Change bolus type: Choose softer solids. • Change bolus size: Reduce size. • Change bolus placement: Utilize lateral bite.

FINDING THE RIGHT POSITION

Feeding therapists are sometimes guilty of focusing so closely on oral and pharyngeal functions that they miss the underlying deficits. In order for the lips and tongue to move efficiently, they must be supported by jaw stability. Jaw stability is dependent on head and neck stability, which in turn is dependent on intact trunk and pelvic stability. We are unlikely, then, to have an impact on the jaw, lips, or tongue with our activities and exercises if we haven't identified and addressed the underlying postural instabilities.

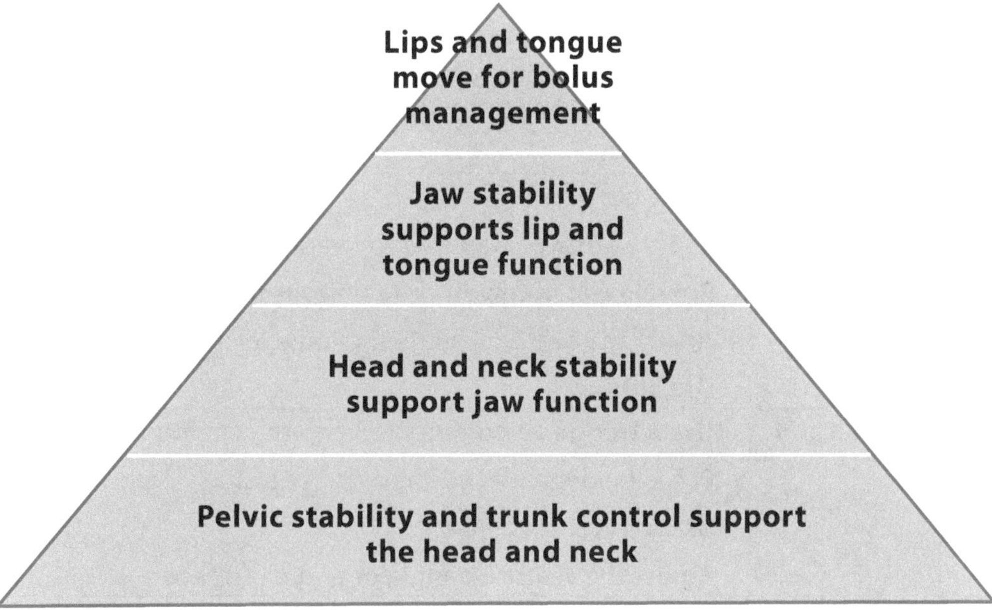

The following table provides some suggestions to help you improve postural stability during feeding.

Suggestion	How to Implement
Improve base of support for feet	• Adjust the seat height so the client's feet are flat on the floor. • Use a footstool or box if the client's feet don't reach the floor. • Use footrests if the client is in a wheelchair.
Improve upright posture	• Avoid seats or stools without a back. • Use a lap belt. • Use a wedge or pommel to keep the client's hips back. • Use a tray.
Improve midline position	• Use a lap belt. • Use a wedge or pommel to keep the client's hips back. • Provide rolled towels or foam rolls for lateral support. • Adjust the seatback angle or angle in space. • Use a tray.
Improve head and neck stability	• Use a wedge or pommel to keep the client's hips back. • Put a headrest on the chair and adjust as necessary. • Use a soft neck pillow. • Adjust the seatback angle or angle in space.
Reduce abnormal tone	• Promote trunk stability via lateral supports. • Adjust the seatback angle or angle in space. • Use a lap belt, wedge, or pommel to keep the client's hips back.
Improve GI comfort	• Keep the abdominal area as open as possible and avoid abdominal compression. • Promote upright posture during and after eating.

Some of our more complicated clients will have multiple positioning concerns that must be met via specialized seating systems, wheelchairs, activity chairs, or specialized strollers. Consider referral to a seating specialist or team to meet the needs of these clients and ensure their safety during feeding.

6

Dealing With "No!": Managing Food Refusal

Food refusal takes many forms in children—omission of entire food groups like fruits or vegetables, restrictions in overall food repertoire, or failure to transition to age-appropriate textures or utensils—and children who don't eat are a significant source of stress for parents and caregivers. Sometimes addressing the underlying respiratory, GI, or motor issues is sufficient to increase volume and variety of intake, but sometimes it's not. Patterns of behavior have been established that need to be changed. Anxiety about new foods or utensils gets in the way of expanding food repertoires. How do we create new, more positive associations around eating?

REDUCING ANXIETY THROUGH FOOD EXPLORATION

Imagine that you couldn't predict how food would feel or taste in your mouth. That every time you took a bite, you were afraid you might gag or choke. That everyone around you was telling you to "just take a bite!" New or unfamiliar foods can be frightening. Food exploration can make them less so by creating familiarity and, perhaps more importantly, predictability. Here are the principles that make up the rules of food exploration:

- You decide what goes in your mouth, and I decide what goes in my mouth.
- There are specific steps to follow when meeting a new food that will make trying it a lot easier.
- Be sure you go through *all* the steps (see the following table). Don't move to bites too quickly.

- Eating is not a spectator sport. If you're at the table, you're part of the exploration team. Nobody just "watches."
- If a step is too challenging, back up to the step before it and spend more time exploring there.
- Avoid words like *good* or *bad*. Instead, focus on the properties of the food.

The table here describes the seven steps involved in food exploration, followed by two food exploration worksheets you can use with children, depending on their age and verbal abilities.

Food Exploration Steps	
1. Use your eyes. Look at the food.	• What colors do you see? • What shapes do you see? • Does it look wet or dry? • Does it look smooth or bumpy? • Does it look the same everywhere? Where is it different? • Does it look like it will crunch? • Does is look soft? • Does it look like foods you've eaten before?
2. Use your fingers and hands to touch the food.	• Does it feel bumpy or smooth? • Is it wet or dry? • Does it feel the same everywhere? • Is it cold or warm? • Were you right about how it would feel? • How do you think it will feel in your mouth? • Does it feel like foods you've eaten before?
3. Use your nose to sniff the food.	• Do you smell anything? • Does it smell strong or not so strong? • Does it smell like anything you know? • How do you think it will taste?

4. Use your lips to "kiss" the food.	• How does it feel on your lips? • Does kissing it feel different than touching it? What's different about it? • Do you taste anything? • Is it wet or dry? • Is it bumpy or smooth? • What's the temperature? • How do you think it will taste?
5. Use your teeth to hold it between your teeth.	• Is it soft or hard? • Can you taste anything? • Do you think that you could bite through it easily or that it would be hard to bite? • Does it feel like something you've tried before? • Can you bite through it (and take it out of your mouth)?
6. Use your tongue to take a lick.	• How does it taste? Is it sweet? Salty? Spicy? • Is it cold or warm? • Does it taste like anything you've tasted before? • Were you right about how it would taste? Is it different than what you expected?
7. Take a tiny "mouse" bite.	• How does it taste? Sweet? Salty? Spicy? • Was your prediction about the taste correct? Was it different from your guess? • Is it easy or hard to chew? • What other foods are like this one?

Client Worksheet (Older/Verbal Child)

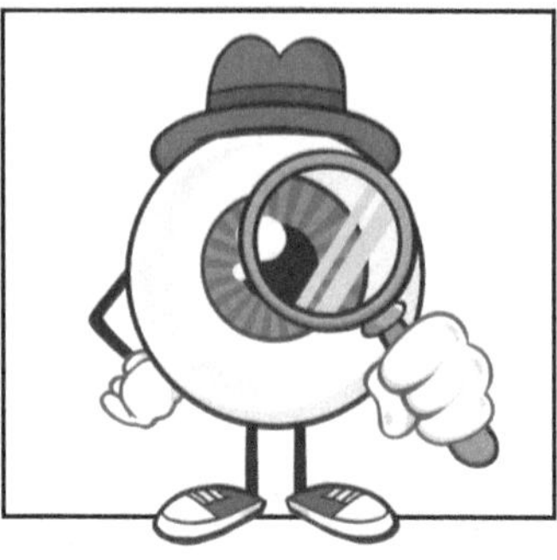

Let's Eat!

Use this worksheet to be a food detective! Use your sense of sight, touch, smell, and taste to describe what this new food is like.

New food:

___

Use your eyes: What colors and shapes do you see?

___

Use your fingers: What does it feel like?

___

Use your nose: What do you smell?

___

Use your lips: How does it feel? What do you think it will taste like?

___

Use your teeth: Is it hard or soft? Can you bite it?

___

Use your tongue: What do you taste?

___

Use your whole mouth to take a small bite: Chew and swallow. Were you right about how it would taste and feel?

___

Client Worksheet (Younger/Nonverbal Child)

Let's Eat!

Can you use these body parts to explore your food?

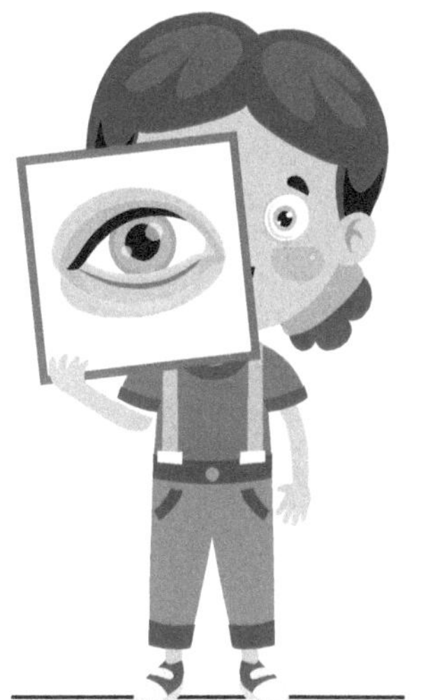
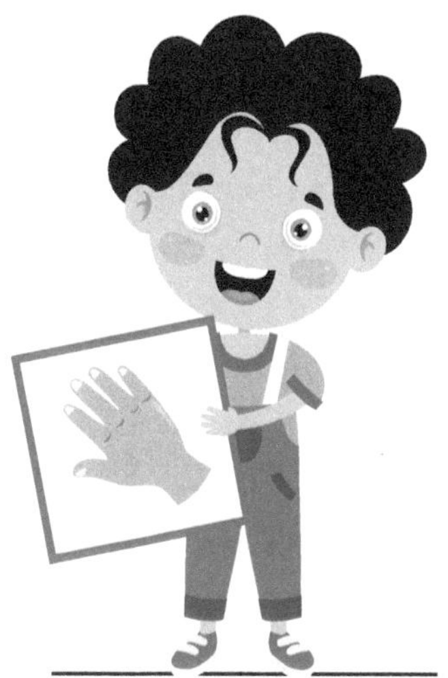
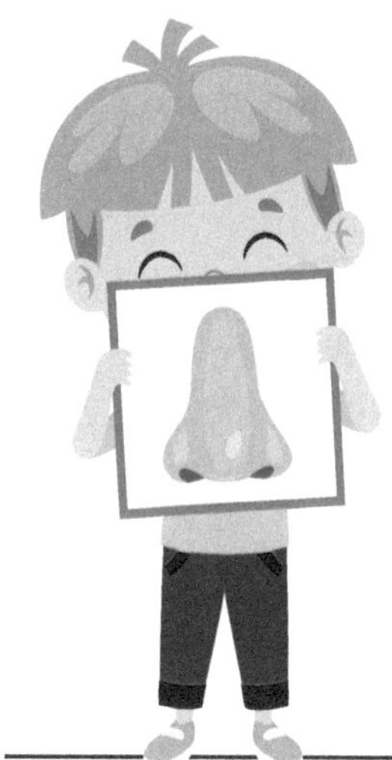

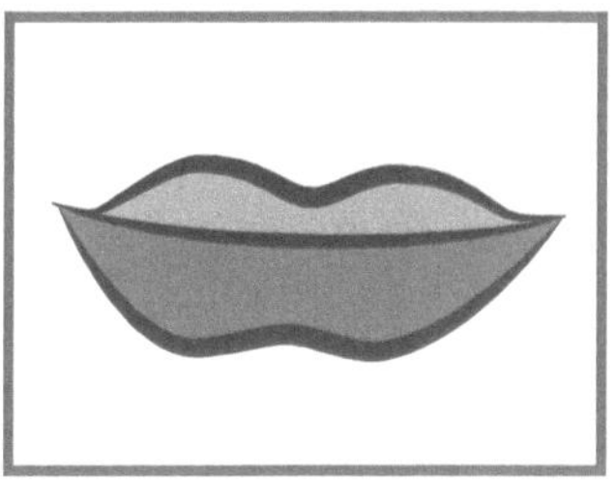
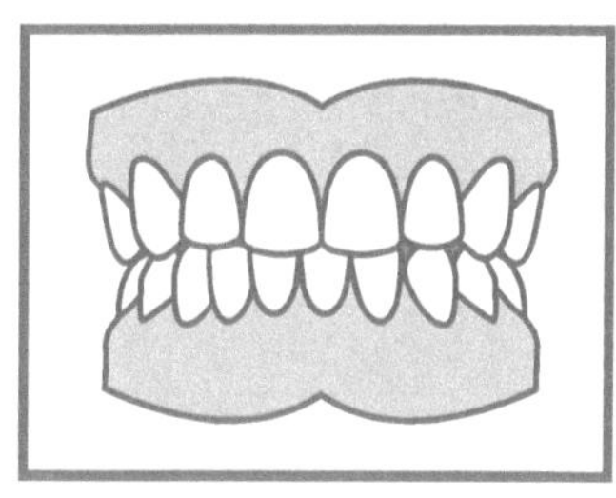
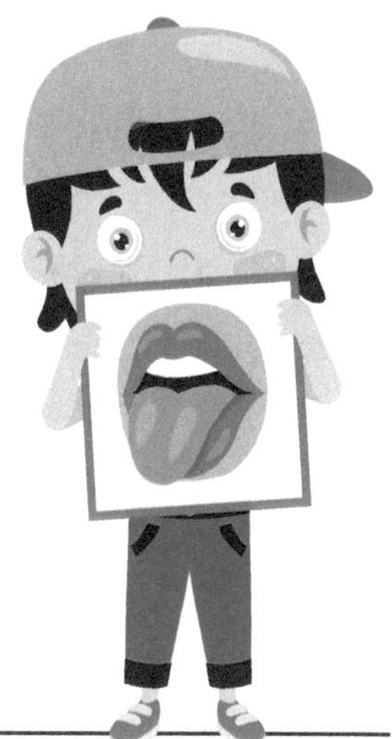

Scripting Success

Social stories were first described by an educator named Carol Gray in the early 1990s as a strategy to improve social skills for children with autism spectrum disorders. In the intervening years, social stories have been used in a variety of contexts and with a variety of children to meet a variety of goals—and feeding is no exception. A *social story* is a short, easy-to-understand, individualized narrative that describes a particular situation or task and suggests an appropriate behavioral response.* Therapists and parents write a story or script for the child that is specific to that child's goals and needs.

A good social story answers the *who*, *what*, *where*, *when*, *why*, and *how* questions for the client as a means of setting expectations, reducing unpredictability, and increasing participation in feeding. A social story contains sentences that describe the situation, what will happen, who will be there, where it will take place, and so on. It also contains coaching sentences that suggest a behavioral response.

Examples of Descriptive Sentences

- Fruits and vegetables make my body grow.
- Some foods are hard for me to eat.
- Sometimes food makes me gag.

Examples of Coaching Sentences

- I can touch the foods to my lips before I eat it.
- I can take a small bite or a big bite.
- I can mix a new food with a food I already like.

We can use social stories very effectively, particularly in the early stages of feeding therapy, to:

- Help our clients understand what feeding therapy is and what the goals are

* Check out www.carolgraysocialstories.com for more information about Carol Gray, the history of social stories, and pertinent research studies.

- Help our clients predict what is going to happen in therapy sessions
- Reduce anxiety about feeding therapy by increasing predictability
- Provide praise and positive feedback

Here are two sample social stories surrounding eating and feeding therapy.

A Story About Eating

People need to eat food.

Food gives us energy to learn, grow, and stay healthy.

Eating food is hard for me sometimes.

I can help my body get ready to eat.

I can take easy breaths.

I can do wall push-ups.

I can squeeze my hands together tightly.

Now I am ready to eat.

A Story About Feeding Therapy

Eating is hard for me.

Food makes me gag sometimes.

Feeding therapy will help me eat more foods.

Feeding therapy will make eating easier for me.

First I touch the food.

Then I smell the food.

Then I touch the food to my lips.

Then I lick the food.

Then I take a very small bite.

Then I take bigger bites.

Practicing with new foods makes them easier to eat.

USING REINFORCEMENT

For many of us, eating has its own rewards: Food is filling, it tastes good, and it's fun. It lets us socialize with our friends or celebrate with our families. It's cake at the birthday party, Sunday dinner with grandparents, turkey at Thanksgiving, candy on Halloween, and hotdogs at a friend's barbecue. But for children with feeding difficulties, eating is not intrinsically rewarding. In fact, it's often exactly the opposite. Eating is frightening. It may cause pain, pressure, or discomfort. It may trigger gagging, choking, or coughing. Therefore, we often need to use reinforcement to create external rewards, particularly at the early stages of feeding therapy.

Targeting Behaviors for Change

When you are working with children who exhibit feeding difficulties, it is important to identify the target behaviors you want to change. What behaviors are interfering with their ability to trial new foods? Are they throwing food? Refusing to participate? Do you have a sense of what the child is trying to communicate with these behaviors? For each of those behaviors, we need to determine two things:

1. What antecedent appears to be triggering those behaviors? A novel food? An unfamiliar utensil? An increase in task demand?
2. What is the response of the feeder or caregiver to the behavior?

Once we've answered these questions, we can examine the results in each category and look for patterns. For example, consider the following scenario that examines the various triggers and responses in relation to a child's feeding behaviors:

Behavior	Antecedent/Trigger	Caregiver Response
Child throws utensil	A spoon with a novel food	Mom offers different food
Child throws food	Non-preferred food	Mom offers different food
Child fusses and cries	Non-preferred food	Dad removes non-preferred food
Child yells "no!"	Unfamiliar food	Dad removes new food

What are the antecedents that trigger the problematic behaviors for this child? As we look at our example, we can see that each of the behaviors is triggered by a novel or non-preferred food or utensil. An analysis of the caregiver responses reveals that each time the child fusses, cries, or refuses, the new or non-preferred item is removed and a more preferred food or utensil is provided. In this case, the parents' behavior (i.e., removing or substituting for non-preferred foods) reinforces the child's behavior (i.e., fussing or refusing in response to non-preferred items), which makes it more likely to happen again. Imagine what happens next: When the parent provides the more familiar or preferred food, it calms the child. Now, the child's behavior (i.e., the cessation of crying) reinforces the parents' behavior (i.e., the provision of more familiar food), which makes it more likely to happen again.

What Is a Reinforcer?

A *reinforcer* is anything (tangible or intangible) that will increase the likelihood that a behavior will occur. You go to work (at least in part) because you get paid. The paycheck is a form of reinforcement because it increases the likelihood that you will continue to go to work each day. Tangible reinforcers include things like toys or screen time, while intangible reinforcers may include praise or attention.

Lots of things have the potential to be good reinforcers, so how do you choose one? You can examine the child's preferences, response to attention or praise, and motivation to accept tokens:

- **Preferences:** Observe the child in play. What does the child like? What would they choose if given the opportunity? Consider toys, games, screen time, and other activities. Parents and other caregivers can often give insight into the child's preferred toys and activities. The taste of a preferred food can be an effective reinforcer for some children as well.
- **Attention or praise:** Is this a child who will work for a "good job" or high five? For many children (and adults as well, of course), the feeling of success can be a powerful reinforcer. Celebrate each touch, lick, and taste.
- **Tokens:** Some children are motivated by a more delayed reward. Each lick or taste earns them a check mark on the page or token in their cup. When they've earned a predetermined number of check marks or tokens, they can turn those in for a larger reward. Ten bites of new food, for example, earns you ten minutes of screen time. Eat your new food at dinner for five days and you've earned a new toy.

A Good Reinforcer...

- Is something the child wants but, more importantly, something the child will *work* for.
- Is something you can control. It's something you can provide and take away.
- Is something the child doesn't otherwise have access to. It's something reserved for feeding activities only.
- Won't work forever. Have backup options when a reinforcer is no longer effective.
- Is easy to understand. Be clear about what the child has to do to earn the reward.
- Doesn't take you away from the table or the task for long.

Positive versus Negative Reinforcement

These can be confusing terms. Try not to think about positive and negative reinforcement in terms of "good" or "bad" but, rather, as mathematical terms. Reinforcement—whether positive or negative—always refers to the way we respond to the desired behavior we're trying to increase. *Positive reinforcement* involves adding something, while *negative reinforcement* involves subtracting something in order to achieve that goal. Consider these examples:

Positive Reinforcement

- During food exploration, your client takes multiple licks of a novel food. You respond with lots of praise and clapping.
- Each time your client takes a "kiss" of a new food, she receives another block to build with.
- Every time your client takes a "mouse" bite of a novel food, this is followed by a bite of a food he likes.

In each case, you're *adding* something to the situation to increase the likelihood that your client will repeat the behavior.

Negative Reinforcement

- Each time your client moves through a step in the food exploration process, she can move away from the table and take a break.
- When your client completes a designated number of bites of his novel food, the session ends.

In each case, you're *subtracting* something from the situation to increase the likelihood that your client will repeat the behavior.

Positive versus Negative Punishment

Punishment is often confused with negative reinforcement, but they are not the same. Remember, reinforcement (whether positive or negative) is the way we respond to a desired behavior to increase its frequency. *Punishment* is the way we respond to an undesirable behavior to decrease its frequency or extinguish it completely. Punishment can be positive and negative as well. As with reinforcement, positive punishment involves adding something, while negative punishment involves subtracting something in response to the undesirable behavior. Consider these examples:

Positive Punishment

- Your client refuses to come to the table. You respond with a verbal prompt, such as "Let's try that again" or "That is an unexpected behavior. What do we do when that happens?"
- Your client says, "That food is yucky!" You respond by saying "Food isn't yucky. Use some describing words to tell me what you noticed when you touched it."

In each case, you're *adding* something to the situation to decrease the likelihood that your client will repeat the behavior.

Negative Punishment

- Your client has been taking mouse bites of an apple but stops participating. You remove the blocks he has been building with until he resumes eating.
- Your client is using words like *gross* or *disgusting* to describe the foods you're exploring. You remove your attention by not responding and ignoring the outbursts.

In each case, you're *subtracting* something from the situation to decrease the likelihood that your client will repeat the behavior.

It's important to have a plan for both reinforcement and punishment. Always be prepared to respond to both the desired behavior and the undesirable behavior.

Matching the Reinforcer to the Task

In order for a reinforcer to be effective, the value of the reinforcer must match the task demand. You may like chocolate, but you wouldn't do your job every day if you were paid in candy bars. Often, when we are having difficulty finding an effective reinforcer, it's because there is a mismatch between the child's perception of the task demand and the value of the reward. And it's the *child's* perception that matters here. Touching or tasting a new food may seem easy enough to us, but it may be incredibly challenging for our clients. As the task demand increases and you move through the stages of food exploration, it is very likely that the value of the reinforcer will have to increase. For example, your client may touch or sniff new foods in exchange for tastes of a preferred food, but they may need something they perceive as more valuable in order to move to licks or bites.

When to Use Reinforcement

When providing reinforcement, it's important to begin by doing so on a schedule. Initially, use *continuous* reinforcement by providing the reinforcer every time the child produces the desired behavior (e.g., touches the food, takes a lick, chews and swallows). As the task progresses, you can fade the reinforcement and implement a more *intermittent* schedule. Intermittent reinforcement can be provided on a fixed schedule (e.g., every five bites) or on a variable schedule.

Continuous reinforcement is helpful in the early stages of therapy because it quickly increases the frequency of the desired response or behavior. Unfortunately, it is difficult to maintain the behavior once the reinforcement is removed, so it is important to begin to move to a more intermittent schedule as soon as the behavior has been established. Intermittent reinforcement may provide a lower response rate, especially initially, but the overall learning is more stable in the long run.

Continuous Reinforcement

- *Every* lick of a novel food is followed by a bite of a preferred food.
- *Each time* the child takes a bite of a new food, they receive a sticker on their sticker chart.

Intermittent Reinforcement

- Every five bites of a novel food is followed by a brief break (fixed schedule).
- Your client is eating a novel, previously non-preferred food. As the child eats, you provide goldfish crackers (preferred food) occasionally (intermittent schedule).

INCORPORATE STRUCTURE

As we discussed, one of the goals of food exploration is to add predictability to a hard-to-predict system. To further that end, we want to build in a predictable structure to our sessions as well. Begin sessions the same way every time—for example, by picking foods to work on, washing your hands, and preparing the table—and incorporate the food exploration steps in a similar sequence each time. End each session the same way too: Review your exploration findings, clean up, and plan for home practice. It is also helpful to structure the language you are using:

- Be calm, clear, and concise: Choose one or two prompts that everyone will use (e.g., "Take a bite").

- Avoid lengthy, multistep directions.
- Avoid coaxing and questions. Say, "It's time to move on to licks" rather than "Are you ready to take a lick?"
- Avoid extraneous demands. Focus only on the task at hand and not on other behaviors.

WHERE TO START? CHOOSING FIRST FOODS

Your client eats only a few foods: chicken nuggets, french fries, waffles, apples with the skin off, grilled cheese sandwiches, and a variety of crackers and cookies. His parents would like him to eat a variety of fruits and vegetables. They would like to be able to eat in a restaurant as a family (other than in fast-food restaurants) and would like him to be able to buy school lunch a few days a week. They would like him to eat what the rest of the family is eating for dinner and to eat at a friend's house on occasion. So...where to start?

First, we need a clear idea of the foods in the current repertoire. We can achieve this goal by asking the client's parents to complete a food inventory or diet diary. (See the examples in chapter 2.) Parents can differentiate between foods the child always eats, sometimes eats, and never eats. Once you have that information, proceed with these steps:

- **Fill in the gaps:** Where are the deficiencies? What's missing from the repertoire? Are there enough protein sources? Enough fruits and vegetables? Calcium and iron sources? Choose a food or foods that will expand the child's diet in one or more of these deficient areas.
- **Consider the family's diet:** What foods do the parents prepare routinely? Are they meat-and-potato eaters or rice-and-bean eaters? Are they vegetarians or grillers? Is pasta a staple? Do they eat salad with every meal? Are they big breakfast eaters or grab-and-go eaters? Choose foods that will fit into the family's regular diet and routines.
- **Use current foods as a bridge to new foods:** Once you've identified the foods that your client eats routinely, think about new foods you can easily add. For example, you can add a small piece of ham between two crackers or in a grilled cheese sandwich. You can include a thin slice of peach on waffles or a cookie. Always start with very small amounts of the novel food, and be sure the child knows what they are eating.

Never hide food. Whenever possible, encourage the child to combine the foods themself so there are no surprises. Make "sandwiches" with small amounts of novel food between two pieces of preferred food. And be sure the child has done some food exploration so the novel food is not completely unfamiliar.

- **Work within the child's sensory system:** What have you learned about this child's sensory system? Is this a child who appears under-responsive and hyposensitive? Does the child look for sensory input by mouthing clothing, toys, and other non-food items? If so, we want to increase this child's volume and variety of oral intake by providing more sensory information in the foods we choose. Consider foods with high flavor—for example, spicy or sour foods—or beverages with carbonation. Crunchy foods may be more easily accepted by this child than softer foods. Cold foods can add input as well.

  In contrast, is this a child who appears to be more over-responsive or hypersensitive? Does this child avoid sensory input? Does this child frequently gag when eating or gag even at the sight or smell of food? If so, this child will need small, measured amounts of input to expand their food repertoire or build volume. Food exploration can be followed by very small bites or tastes of novel foods. Consider foods that have more neutral tastes, and avoid strong flavors. Choose foods that the child can eat at room temperature, and avoid foods that are too hot or cold.

  Food choice alone, however, may not meet the sensory needs of every child. We may need to incorporate some calming or alerting activities before or during feeding, depending on whether the child is over- or under-responsive. For example, an under-responsive child may need to get up from the table to move around at times and engage in activities that will continue to alert their system. Swinging or spinning activities may provide the additional input that this child needs to return to the table and continue eating. In contrast, an over-responsive child may require calming activities prior to eating and intermittently throughout the meal.

SMALL BITES ARE BIG STEPS

Parents often ask, "How much should my child be eating?" In this "super-sized" world we live in, it is easy to incorporate an exaggerated sense of portion size into our expectations. In fact, children may require smaller portions than we think! The American Academy of Pediatrics recommends the following serving sizes:*

Serving Size Recommendation	1 to 6 Years	7 to 10 Years	Daily Servings
Fruits	¼ cup canned or ½ piece fresh	½ cup canned or 1 piece fresh	2–3 servings/day
Vegetables	¼ cup	½ cup	2–3 servings/day
Grains	½ slice bread ¼ to ⅓ cup cereal, rice, or pasta 2–4 crackers	1 slice bread ½ cup cereal, rice, or pasta 4–5 crackers	6–11 servings/day
Meat/protein	1 oz meat or tofu ¼ to ⅓ cup beans ½ to 1 egg	2–3 oz meat or tofu ½ cup beans 1–2 eggs	2 servings/day
Dairy	½ cup milk ½ to 1 oz cheese ⅓ to ½ cup yogurt	1 cup milk 1 oz cheese ¾ to 1 cup yogurt	2–3 servings/day

For children with feeding difficulties, it is often better to keep your expectations low. Too much food on the plate, particularly if it is a novel or non-preferred food, can seem overwhelming and may result in continued food refusals. Present small amounts, especially at the early stages of therapy. In other words, place one slice of carrot on the plate instead of several whole carrots, or a small piece of chicken rather than the whole chicken breast.

It is also helpful to remember that younger children regulate their appetite differently than older children and adults. Rather than eating a consistent amount at breakfast, lunch, and dinner, they are more likely to eat consistent amounts over a 24- to 48-hour period. In other words, they may eat a large breakfast and then eat very little for lunch or dinner. Or they may not eat much throughout the day until dinner and then eat a larger amount. This variability is not a cause for alarm but is, in fact, very normal.

* For more information, check out www.healthychildren.org.

AVOIDING THE GAG

Children with feeding difficulties often come to us with a history of unpleasant experiences with food. They have learned that food makes them feel bad. They understandably have a great deal of anxiety about eating. Gagging and other unpleasant responses can reinforce the idea that food is bad and something to be avoided. So how do we reduce gagging and limit its interference as we complete our food exploration activities?

- **Keep the bite size small:** Limit the sensory input by initially keeping bites and sips small.
- **Provide simultaneous pleasant sensory experiences:** Mask the non-preferred taste or smell by pairing the new food with a preferred, more familiar food.
- **Place foods and utensils on the side of the mouth:** Avoid the gag response by placing food and utensils laterally on the side teeth.
- **Breathe:** Interrupt the gag by blowing out through pursed lips as if you were blowing out a candle.

EATING EVERYWHERE: TRANSITIONING TO HOME, SCHOOL, AND THE COMMUNITY

As involved as all this may seem, getting children to eat new foods in the therapeutic environment of the clinic is really the easy part. The difficult part is carrying over those skills to a variety of other feeding environments. We all eat in a variety of places with a variety of people: family dinners at home, a quick snack in the car, lunch in the cafeteria at school, or supper at a friend's house. We need a plan to assist children in transitioning their new eating skills to a wider range of places. To do so, we can practice eating new foods in a number of places, set scheduled practice times, institute family mealtimes, and get kids in the kitchen.

Practice New Foods in a Number of Places

It is never too early to begin practicing outside of the therapy environment: at home, school, grandma's house, or daycare. Have the child take whatever food they've been practicing in the clinic home with them for more practice. The simple act of carrying that bag of apple slices home or to daycare can serve as a bridge to eating in new environments. Practice may involve only touches, sniffs, or licks in the initial stages, but it is important to incorporate a variety of feeding environments and partners as soon as possible. The following checklists, logs, and visual schedules can be helpful at this stage to keep everybody on track.

Child Worksheet

Food Log I

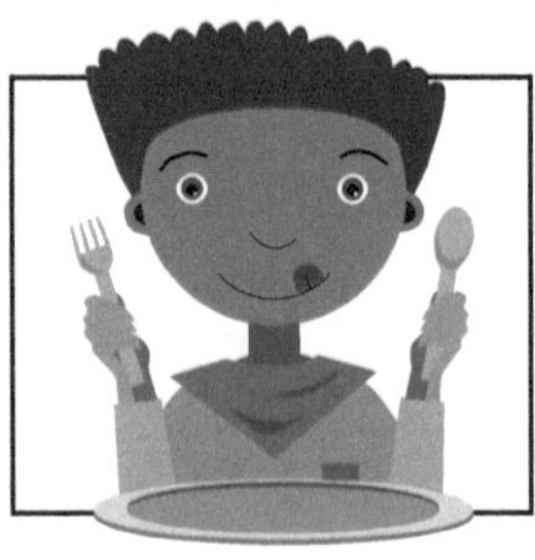

Use this log to record all the new foods you've tried this week. Place a check mark in the box to indicate if you licked, bit, or swallowed that food.

Day	Food(s)	Licked	Bit	Swallowed
Sunday	______________	☐	☐	☐
Monday	______________	☐	☐	☐
Tuesday	______________	☐	☐	☐
Wednesday	______________	☐	☐	☐
Thursday	______________	☐	☐	☐
Friday	______________	☐	☐	☐
Saturday	______________	☐	☐	☐

Child Worksheet

Food Log II

Practice what we learned in feeding therapy. Start small and make your bites bigger and bigger. How big can you make them?

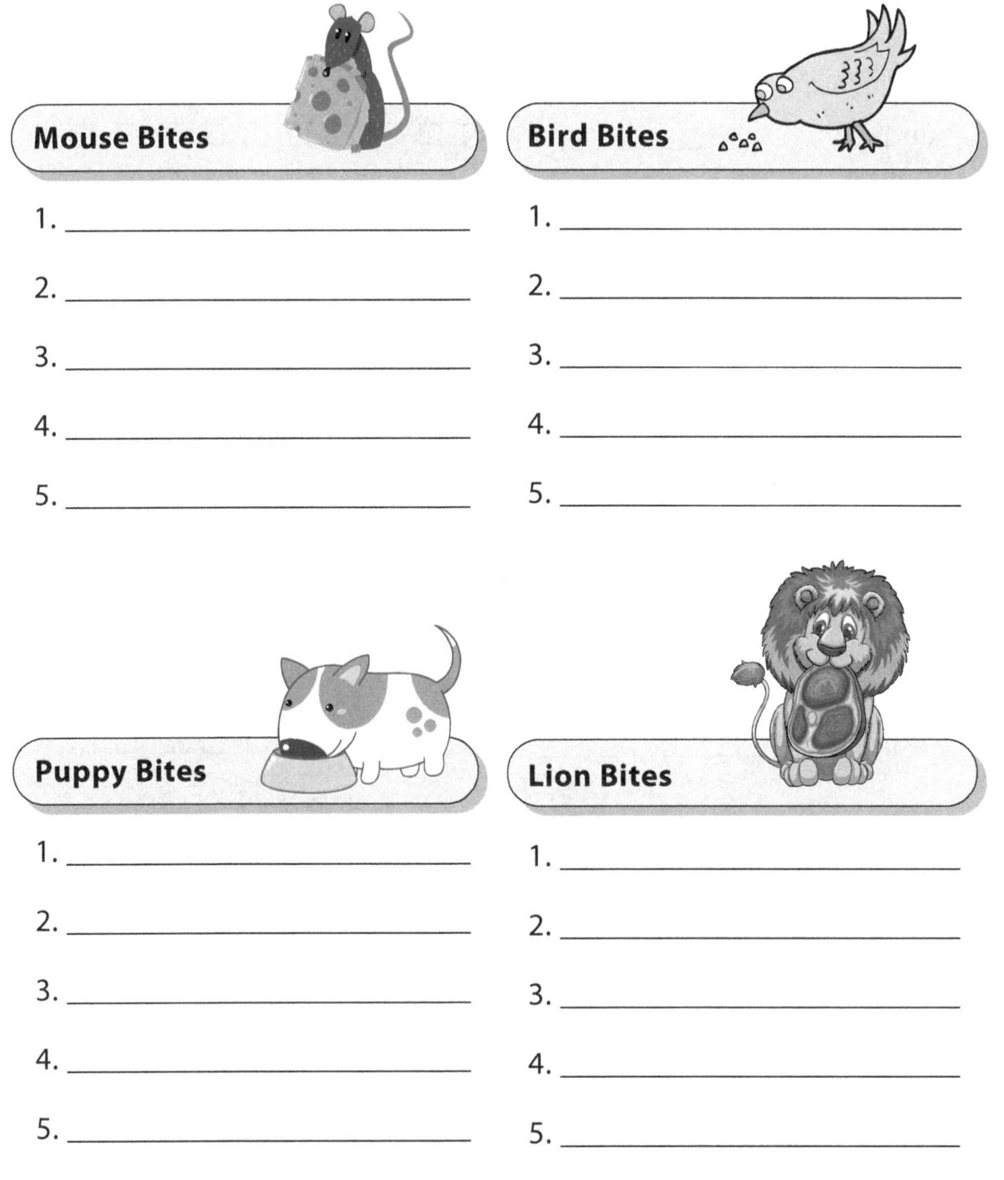

Mouse Bites

1. ______________________
2. ______________________
3. ______________________
4. ______________________
5. ______________________

Bird Bites

1. ______________________
2. ______________________
3. ______________________
4. ______________________
5. ______________________

Puppy Bites

1. ______________________
2. ______________________
3. ______________________
4. ______________________
5. ______________________

Lion Bites

1. ______________________
2. ______________________
3. ______________________
4. ______________________
5. ______________________

Child Worksheet

Food Log III

Use this log to record all the new foods you've tried **at home** this week. Place a check mark to indicate how many bites of the food you took!

Day	Food	Number of Bites
Sunday	______________	☐ ☐ ☐ ☐ ☐ ☐ ☐ ☐ ☐ ☐
Monday	______________	☐ ☐ ☐ ☐ ☐ ☐ ☐ ☐ ☐ ☐
Tuesday	______________	☐ ☐ ☐ ☐ ☐ ☐ ☐ ☐ ☐ ☐
Wednesday	______________	☐ ☐ ☐ ☐ ☐ ☐ ☐ ☐ ☐ ☐
Thursday	______________	☐ ☐ ☐ ☐ ☐ ☐ ☐ ☐ ☐ ☐
Friday	______________	☐ ☐ ☐ ☐ ☐ ☐ ☐ ☐ ☐ ☐
Saturday	______________	☐ ☐ ☐ ☐ ☐ ☐ ☐ ☐ ☐ ☐

Child Worksheet

Food Log IV

Use this log to record all the new foods you've tried **at school** this week. Place a check mark to indicate how many bites of the food you took!

Day	Food	Number of Bites
Monday	____________	☐ ☐ ☐ ☐ ☐ ☐ ☐ ☐ ☐ ☐
Tuesday	____________	☐ ☐ ☐ ☐ ☐ ☐ ☐ ☐ ☐ ☐
Wednesday	____________	☐ ☐ ☐ ☐ ☐ ☐ ☐ ☐ ☐ ☐
Thursday	____________	☐ ☐ ☐ ☐ ☐ ☐ ☐ ☐ ☐ ☐
Friday	____________	☐ ☐ ☐ ☐ ☐ ☐ ☐ ☐ ☐ ☐

Getting the Practice Done

As with most therapy programs, adherence outside of the therapy setting can be a challenge. To facilitate better adherence (from both the child and the parents), we can establish a plan, not just for the practice but for *completion* of the practice. Discuss where and when the practice could reasonably take place. Is breakfast just too hectic? Then maybe dinner is a better time to practice. Is there just no time at daycare? Then let's practice at home. Does the child do better when other children are around? Then perhaps snack time at school is best.

Incorporate both individual and group practice opportunities given that each provide different types of benefits. A one-to-one practice session provides the child with focused attention, prompts, and cues without distractions, whereas a group practice session (e.g., family mealtime, school snack) provides the benefits of peer modeling and gives the child opportunities to participate in the social aspects of eating.

In addition to a plan for where and when, be clear about *how much* practice should occur. Every day? Five days a week? Ten bites? A whole apple? Two foods? If you've been using reinforcement, then include that in your plan as well. What reinforcement will be used at home? At school? When will the reinforcement be provided? Involve the child in these discussions whenever possible. Providing the child with some control over the *where*, *when*, and *what* of the practice increases the likelihood that they will actually do the practice.

Institute Family Mealtimes

The research is clear: Families that eat together on a regular basis have children with better nutrition, healthier relationships and social skills, and less problematic adolescent behaviors, like drug and nicotine use. But you may not know that there are many desirable outcomes associated with family mealtimes related to feeding as well. In fact, family mealtimes can:

- Decrease "picky" eating (Cole et al., 2018; Verhage et al., 2018)
- Increase fruit and vegetable consumption (Caldwell et al., 2018)
- Increase the intake of healthy foods, like proteins, grains, and vegetables (Lee et al., 2014)

Here are some strategies to help your clients implement successful family mealtimes:

- Have everybody eat the same thing, including some preferred foods and some new foods.
- Include some child-friendly foods that are easy to eat and cut into small pieces.
- Allow every family member the opportunity to choose foods sometimes.
- Include at least one preferred food at each meal.
- Get children involved in pre- and post-meal rituals, like setting the table, preparing the meal, and cleaning up.
- Praise appropriate behaviors at mealtimes.
- Let the small stuff go (e.g., ignore fidgeting, messiness, complaining)
- Embrace that it might be messy!

Get Kids in the Kitchen

Children are more likely to try foods they helped make, so we want to get kids in the kitchen as soon as possible. Many children like to help in the kitchen because it makes them feel grown up, and it's fun too. The table here provides some suggestions you can use to help kids of various ages assist in the kitchen, and it is followed by an educational handout you can give parents and caregivers regarding mealtime "dos" and "don'ts."

Young children (2 to 4 years) can:	Older children (4 to 5 years and older) can:
• Put things on the table • Tear up lettuce, snap green beans • Make "art" with pieces of fruit or vegetables • Rinse foods in water • Scoop foods onto a plate • Stir batter in a bowl • Peel bananas, oranges • Help with measuring • Put meat and cheese on bread for a sandwich • Put things in the trash after eating	• Help with meal planning • Crack eggs into a bowl • Use an eggbeater • Make sandwiches and salads • Cut foods • Use a cookie cutter • Open cans • Cook and bake with assistance or supervision from a grown-up • Clear the table • Put things in the dishwasher

Parent/Caregiver Handout

Mealtime Dos and Don'ts

Few things are more frustrating than when your child doesn't eat. Here are a few tips to make eating easier for them… and you!

DO…

- ☐ Have meals at regular times
- ☐ Include pre- and post-meal activities
- ☐ Use a visual schedule
- ☐ Praise your child
- ☐ Provide age-appropriate portions
- ☐ Let the small stuff go (it's going to be messy!)
- ☐ Celebrate small victories
- ☐ Lower your expectations (small tastes are big victories)
- ☐ Save liquid supplements (such as PediaSure®) for the end of the day to increase appetite

DON'T…

- ☐ Insist on an empty plate
- ☐ Serve food in or from commercial containers
- ☐ Allow liquids before eating
- ☐ Force feed
- ☐ Serve the same thing all the time
- ☐ Expect your child to eat something you're not going to eat
- ☐ Hide food

7

Tube Feeding: Who, When, and for How Long?

For some of our clients, eating by mouth is simply not safe or even possible. For these children, non-oral or alternative nutrition and hydration (ANH), is utilized. You may also hear or see the term *enteral nutrition*, which is a broader term used to refer to methods of feeding that utilize the GI tract. This clearly could include oral feeding, but sometimes enteral feeding is used to refer specifically to tube feeding. This book differentiates enteral feeding, which uses the GI tract, from parenteral feeding, which delivers nutrition directly into a vein. Whenever feasible, enteral feeding is preferable.

WHAT DO WE NEED TO KNOW ABOUT FEEDING TUBES?

Tube Types

Tube feeding can be done in several different ways. In this section, I will talk about the different tube types that may be used, the different schedules implemented, and the challenges associated with tube feeding, both medical and practical.

Enteral tube feeding is nutrition that is delivered directly into the GI system:

- **Orogastric tube (OG tube):** The feeding tube enters through the mouth, through the esophagus, and into the stomach.
- **Nasogastric tube (NG tube):** The feeding tube is passed through the nose, through the esophagus, and into the stomach. A nasoduodenal tube continues through the stomach and into the duodenum, which is the beginning of the small intestine, while a nasojejunal tube continues farther through the small intestine into the jejunum.

- **Gastrostomy tube (G-tube):** The feeding tube is surgically placed through the stomach and delivers nutrition directly into the stomach. You may also see the term *percutaneous endoscopic gastrostomy (PEG)*, which refers to the manner in which the tube is placed (i.e., endoscopically instead of surgically).
- **Jejunostomy tube (J-tube):** The feeding tube is surgically placed into the jejunum, which is the lower part of the intestine, and delivers nutrition into the jejunum.
- **Gastro-jejunal tube (G-J tube):** These tubes have two ports: a G-port and a J-port. Initially, a G-tube is placed and then extended and connected to the jejunum via a long tube. The J-port opening is typically used for nutrition, while the G-port opening is used for medications or to vent air. In some children, the G-port may be used for nutrition as well.

In contrast to enteral feeding, parenteral nutrition is delivered into the bloodstream and bypasses the GI system:

- **Peripheral parenteral nutrition (PPN):** Fluids are delivered through a catheter inserted into a vein. Intravenous nutrition is typically limited to sugars (glucose), and because of the low concentration, smaller veins can be used.
- **Total parenteral nutrition (TPN):** Fluids that contain sugars (but also potentially proteins, fats, electrolytes, vitamins, and minerals) are delivered through a central venous catheter. There are different types of ports and catheters than can be used, depending on the type of nutrition and the location of the port. You may hear the terms *central venous catheter*, *central line*, *peripherally inserted central catheter (PICC) line*, or *Hickman catheter*. These are all examples of TPN delivery systems.

As the following table illustrates, each of these nutrition delivery methods has its advantages and challenges.

Method	Advantages	Challenges
OG tube	• Reduced nasal irritation or sinusitis compared to nasal tubes	• Short-term use only • Generally used in sedated clients and thus not for home use • Potential for dental damage
NG (or ND or NJ) tube	• Easy to place and replace (does not require surgery or sedation for placement) • Suitable for short-term use	• Significant risk of reflux • Some potential for discomfort (the tube must be taped to the face to keep it in place) • Visible • Can be easily pulled out by the child • Requires frequent replacement • Can cause gagging in some children
G-tube	• Easily replaced at home • Provides options for nutrition delivery type and schedule • Can use real food or blended diets • Some potential for reflux but less than with NG tubes	• Requires surgical/endoscopic placement • Potential for irritation or infection at the tube site • Does not prevent reflux or aspiration of reflux
J-tube	• Decreases risk of reflux and aspiration of reflux	• Requires medical procedure for replacement • Requires a pump and continuous feeding
G-J tube	• Same as for G-tubes and J-ports	• Same as for G-tubes and J-ports
PPN/TPN	• Bypasses the GI system for clients with non-functional GI tracts • PPN is helpful for supplemental hydration or provision of electrolytes	• Potential for occlusion (blockage or clogging), clotting, and infection • Potential for burning and swelling at the insertion site • Requires an infusion pump • Requires close medical monitoring

Feeding Tube Schedules

There are two different types of tube feeding schedules: continuous feeding and intermittent or bolus feeding. *Continuous feeding* is done in small amounts continuously over several hours. Continuous feeding requires that the tube is attached to a pump, which can limit mobility in some children. For fragile, medically complicated infants and children, continuous feeds are sometimes better tolerated because they require less energy expenditure. Clients with respiratory impairments, in particular, may benefit from continuous feeding as a strategy for conserving energy.

Bolus feeding, in contrast, provides larger amounts of liquid (or puree in some cases) at intervals throughout the day. Bolus feeding can be done by hand with a syringe or via gravity feeding (i.e., the formula is contained in a syringe or bag and allowed to drip into the tube). Pumps are sometimes used if the bolus needs to be administered more slowly. Bolus feeding can normalize hunger-satiation signals and is an important tool when the child is ready to begin weaning from the tube.

Bolus feeds allow us to simulate a more typical mealtime schedule, but not all children can tolerate bolus feeds. For those children who require slower nutrition delivery, continuous feeding or a combination of bolus and continuous feeding is often recommended. Many children receive bolus feeds throughout the day and continuous feeds overnight while sleeping. It is important to understand a client's bolus feeding schedule—and why they are on that schedule—as we begin to work toward weaning them from the tube. I will discuss weaning in more detail later in this chapter.

Feeding Tube Formulas

There are various types of feeding tube formulas available, depending on the client's needs. Your child's dietician or physician will choose a formula based on the child's medical condition, GI function, and known or suspected allergies. The following table describes several common formulas.

Formula Type	Indications	Composition	Examples
Standard formulas	Recommended for babies and children with normally functioning GI systems	• Nutritionally complete (i.e., contain proteins, carbohydrates, fats, vitamins, and minerals) • Can be milk or soy based	PediaSure® Similac®
Hydrolyzed (or peptide) formulas	Recommended for clients with known or suspected allergies or intolerances or with GI dysfunction	• Nutritionally complete • Proteins are partially broken down for easier digestion • Some contain cow's milk protein	Peptamen Junior®
Elemental (or extensively hydrolyzed) formulas	Recommended for clients with significant GI dysfunction, food allergies, or history of formula intolerance	• Nutritionally complete • Proteins and fats are completely broken down into amino acids • Hypoallergenic	EleCare® Neocate®
Blenderized (blended) formulas	Recommended for clients with normally functioning GI systems and are helpful when preparing for tube weaning	• Contain real food	Compleat® Pediatric Real Food Blends™ Nourish®
Specialized formulas	Recommended for specific medical and health conditions, including seizure disorders and kidney disease	• Formulated to meet specific dietary needs	KetoCal® Renalcal®

TUBE FEEDING CHALLENGES

Tube feeding is not without its difficulties. We know that children with feeding tubes are at risk for infection or tissue breakdown at the tube site, tube blockages or dislocations, and perforations. Unfortunately, these complications often result in visits to the emergency room or, in more severe cases, hospital admissions (Goldberg et al., 2010; Goldin et al., 2016). It is a common misconception that tube feeding eliminates aspiration risk given that the presence of a feeding tube in children who are known to aspirate may actually increase hospitalization for pulmonary illnesses (McSweeney et al., 2015). The tube does not eliminate the risk of aspiration of saliva and may increase reflux and aspiration of reflux. Not surprisingly, parents also report that tube feeding is more care-intensive as well.

There are three challenges in particular that feeding therapists need to be aware of, seeing as they have the potential to impact our attempts to decrease feeding-tube dependency and wean clients from the tube: reflux, volume intolerance, and overnight feeding.

1. **Reflux:** The presence of an NG tube or a G-tube can increase reflux episodes and therefore increase the potential for aspiration of reflux. Upright positioning during feeding and for 30 minutes or more afterward is critical to reflux management in tube-fed children. If nighttime feedings are provided, be sure that the head of the bed is elevated and that the child can maintain a semi-upright position during the feeding.

2. **Volume intolerance:** Some children can tolerate tube feeding in small volumes or at a slow rate only. There are many potential reasons for this, including food allergies or sensitivities, slowed gastric emptying, and difficulties with absorption. Children who were poor oral feeders prior to their feeding tube insertion may not be used to the amount or density of calories now being provided through the tube. GI problems like reflux disease and constipation can also contribute to volume intolerance.

   What does volume intolerance look like? Children may vomit during or after feedings. They may gag or retch. They may experience bloating and gas pain. In these cases, we can take the following steps to improve volume tolerance:

   - Working with the child's physician and dietician, we can adjust the feeding schedule or the formula itself. Children with volume intolerance can benefit from a slower rate of feeding or from a less concentrated formula. Some children benefit from more free water through the tube to improve constipation and gastric motility, and you should discuss this with the dietician or physician on your team as well.

- Improving overall gastric motility through medical management of the reflux or constipation can also help with volume intolerance. (See chapter 3 for a full discussion of management of GI issues.)
- For children with a gastric port (i.e., G-tube or G-J tube), venting excess air out of the stomach by opening the port can help make the child more comfortable and improve volume tolerance. Gently massaging the stomach or raising the child's legs to the chest can help vent air out of the stomach through the port as well.
- Blended diets (i.e., real food through the tube) can help normalize gastric function and help with volume tolerance.

3. **Overnight feeding:** Some children cannot tolerate exclusive bolus feeding and require continuous feeding for some or all of their intake. For a number of reasons, some of that feeding is often accomplished at night, when the child is asleep. For some children, there is simply not enough time during the day to complete the intake because the flow rate is so slow. In other cases, it is more convenient to run the feeding at night because it will not interfere with the child's mobility.

   However, there are some implications to nighttime feeding that we should be aware of. Reflux and aspiration of reflux risks increase with nighttime feedings because the child is not awake or alert and is often in a more reclined position. Elevating the head of the bed is essential during nighttime feedings for this reason. There is also some evidence to suggest that asking the body to digest food continuously throughout the night changes circadian rhythms. It is not clear what, if any, effect this has on overall health and immune system functioning, so we should monitor our clients carefully for signs of nighttime discomfort or sleep disruptions.

FEEDING TUBE DEPENDENCY

What Is Feeding Tube Dependency?

Perhaps the most persistent and long-lasting challenge associated with tube feeding is feeding tube dependency. Krom et al. (2017) define feeding tube dependency as long-term feeding tube use that results in one or more of the following:

- Active refusal to eat or drink
- Inability to learn to eat or drink
- Lack of motivation to eat or drink
- Lack of development of feeding skills

Children with feeding tube dependency remain tube fed well beyond the intended period of tube use and may avoid food, exhibit agitation or other maladaptive behaviors associated with feeding activities, and demonstrate anxiety or over-responsiveness to eating activities, including gagging or vomiting. Feeding tube dependency can be stressful for parents as well. They often feel powerless in the face of the child who absolutely refuses to eat. Unfortunately, many doctors don't recognize feeding tube dependency as a problem. "She gets what she needs through the tube, right?" is a common response parents and feeding therapists receive when they express concerns about difficulties with oral feeding.

What causes feeding tube dependency in children? Rarely does a single experience or medical condition result in tube dependence. These are children who have experienced uncomfortable and often painful procedures. They've been poked, tubed, moved, and injected repeatedly, and they have learned that many of these experiences are outside of their control. The thing they can control, however, is what goes in (or doesn't go in) their mouths. In fact, we often see regression in oral feeding following a hospitalization or procedure, even one unrelated to the feeding tube or oral feeding.

Prolonged feeding tube use can also interfere with the child's hunger-satiation cycle and effectively mute their hunger signals. Many tube-dependent children have never had the opportunity to regulate their own hunger or satiety signals because of their medical conditions. In addition, the child may have missed opportunities to develop feeding skills due to medical conditions or complications. Or they may have learned that eating results in negative experiences for them, including gagging, vomiting, or retching.

Not all feeding tube dependency looks the same. Some children may be completely indifferent to oral feeding. Others may actively avoid oral intake or find it aversive. Some may exhibit interest in eating, but their volume of oral intake is low and not sufficient to maintain nutrition or hydration.

For other children, oral feeding may be unsafe or impossible given their dysphagia or other medical conditions.

Can Tube Dependency Be Prevented?

The answer is maybe. There are some things the team can do when the tube is placed and as tube feedings progress, but some babies and children are simply so medically compromised that efforts to decrease tube dependency take a back seat to their other medical needs.

What *can* we do?

1. **Normalize tube feeds:** Cuddle the baby close, in the same way you would during bottle-feeding or breastfeeding. Complete tube feedings during family mealtimes, at the kitchen table with friends, or in the rec room with the cousins at Auntie's house—wherever and whenever other people eat and drink. This can be a problem in school settings as tube feedings are often provided by the school nurse in the nursing office. It simply may not be feasible to provide tube feedings in the classroom or cafeteria. Instead, determine what amount and type of oral intake is safe, and encourage school staff to provide that during snack or lunch breaks.

2. **Establish mealtime routines:** To the extent possible, provide nutrition through the tube on an age-appropriate feeding schedule. This means moving to bolus feeding and away from continuous feeding as soon as the child is ready. However, this should not be done at the expense of comfort. If bolus feeds are making the child uncomfortable, causing bloating or pain, or increasing reflux or constipation, they won't help us in our efforts to reduce tube dependency. In fact, they may be making things worse.

3. **Encourage oral intake whenever possible:** Encourage the child to interact with foods in whatever way they would like. Provide the child with opportunities to touch, smell, and taste the foods. If oral feeding has been determined to be safe only for certain food types or textures, have those available at each meal so the child can safely participate in the mealtime. Give the child opportunities to participate in family meal preparation too. Meal preparation gives children experience with touching, smelling, and even tasting foods.

4. **Avoid aversive input and experiences:** Encourage, but never force, interaction with foods. Be sure that the child is followed by a

gastroenterologist and perhaps an allergist as well. We want to identify and manage any underlying medical condition, like constipation or food allergies, that may be causing pain or discomfort during eating.

5. **Use mealtime language:** Rather than using terms like *bolus* or *G-tube*, say to the child, "It's time to eat," "Let's have a drink," or "You must be hungry." Language matters, and we can use it to send the message that eating is *not* a medical procedure. In fact, it's a natural process that everybody does (although in different ways), and it's also something that families and friends do together.

6. **Provide oral play and oral stimulation:** Create opportunities for positive experiences around the mouth. For infants, non-nutritive sucking on a pacifier can facilitate a calm state and promote readiness for oral feeding. As babies get older, we want to continue to provide positive input around the mouth. What is pleasurable for this child? For some children, it might be vibration; for others, cold temperatures; and for others, texture. Parents often ask what the right chew or teething toy is for their child, and the answer is, whichever ones they like, seek out, and will accept for more than just a few seconds.

FEEDING TUBE WEANING

Weaning a baby or child from a tube can be a lengthy process, particularly for children with long-term tube dependence. No single feeding therapist can (or should) wean a baby or child by themself. Successful weaning requires the work of a team that includes the feeding therapist, the physician, the dietician, the parents, and the child.

How do we know when and where to start? As with any transition, we look for readiness signs.

Readiness Signs

To determine whether a child is ready to transition to oral feeding, it can help to ask yourself these questions:

- What is the reason the tube was originally placed? Has that issue been resolved? If not, a full wean from the tube is unlikely.
- Is the child medically stable? Nutritionally stable? Weaning is likely to compromise the child's nutritional status (at least temporarily), so the child must be able to sustain a period of no weight gain, or even weight loss, without significant medical or nutritional compromise.

- Does the child have sufficient oral motor and pharyngeal swallow function to support oral feeding? Full oral feeding is not feasible if the child is unable to swallow without aspirating or chew without risk of choking.
- Are the parents ready? Do they have the practical resources they need? The emotional resources? New oral feeders often require substantially more supervision, assistance, and time.

Once you've determined that weaning is feasible from a practical, medical, and nutritional standpoint, it's time to start to make the transition to oral feeding. Weaning can be challenging, particularly for children with long-term tube dependence, so let's discuss some tools and strategies to help us meet the challenge.

Hunger Manipulation

Hunger seems simple, right? Your stomach is empty, and your body lets you know it needs to eat by growling at you. In reality, it's actually a more complicated combination of stomach contractions, hormonal signals, and neural transmissions between the gut and the brain. While hunger is the physical signal that we need to eat, appetite is a desire to eat, often triggered by the sight, smell, or sometimes thought of foods. When your stomach is "growling," ghrelin hormones are stimulating gastric motility and contractions of the stomach muscles. That's hunger. When someone offers you chocolate and you take it even though you've just finished dinner, that's appetite. When blood sugar levels are low and your stomach feels empty, that's hunger. When you stop into that bakery because the cinnamon rolls smell so good, that's appetite. Hunger and appetite interact to impact volume and variety of intake.

Hunger is perhaps the most critical component of tube weaning. Why would we expect a child to eat if they are getting everything they need (nutritionally) through the tube? In order to see an increase in oral intake, we have to reduce the calories going through the tube. While this idea makes sense physiologically, it does raise questions and concerns: Will the child lose weight? Become malnourished? Feel uncomfortable? How do we manipulate hunger (and perhaps appetite too) to work to our advantage as we move children from tubes to oral feeding? To address these issues, we can focus on the feeding schedule, caloric intake, and medication:

- **Feeding schedule:** Working with the child's dietician or gastroenterologist (whoever is providing medical management of the tube feeding), arrange the feeding schedule to promote hunger. In other words, the child should have periods each day during which they do not receive nutrition via the tube in order to promote hunger.

- **Caloric intake:** The number of calories being provided via the tube should be reduced as much as possible, as quickly as possible, and (of course) as safely as possible. Weight loss is likely, particularly with rapid weans, and the child's weight should be monitored closely. You should discuss specific parameters for each child with the child's physician, but in general, weight loss should not be more than 10 percent of the initial weight. In some cases, children are nutritionally "primed"—in other words, calories have been adjusted to promote weight gain—before beginning the weaning process in order to provide extra weight as a safety net of sorts once the weaning process begins. During rapid weans (described later in this chapter), the child will receive weight checks daily, or at a minimum every other day, to monitor weight loss and alert the team if the child nears the parameter set for discontinuation. More gradual weans also require regular weight checks but not at the same frequency.
- **Medication:** Although the use of medication to stimulate appetite and facilitate tube weaning has not been well studied, some physicians prescribe appetite stimulants for children with feeding disorders. Typically, medications such as cyproheptadine or megestrol are utilized, though antianxiety medications are occasionally used to help reduce the fear associated with oral intake. Medications always have potential side effects, and appetite stimulants often have anticholinergic effects, so consider medication as a last resort in the weaning process.

Gut Priming

As we work to transition children from tube to oral feeding, we need to normalize gut functions. We accomplish this through gut priming—in other words, by normalizing tube feeding as much as possible. As discussed earlier, we can accomplish this by providing nutrition through the tube that mirrors the mealtime schedule as closely as possible. We also have to think about the formula that's going through the tube. Moving away from predigested, hydrolyzed, or extensively hydrolyzed formulas to standard or blended (blenderized) formulas challenges the digestive system in a more normal way.

However, our most effective tool for gut priming is *variety*. Humans rarely eat the same things meal after meal, day after day. Today we may eat eggs and bacon for breakfast, a sandwich at lunch, and meat and potatoes for dinner, but tomorrow it may be pancakes in the morning, a salad for lunch, and pasta for dinner. This variety is one of the things that helps create a diverse microbiome that is so critical to normal digestive and immune system functioning. One way families provide this variety in tube-fed children is by using real foods through the tube.

Blenderized (Blended) Diets

We can include real food through the tube in two ways: through commercially available, pre-measured real-food formulas or through homemade liquid and puree mixtures. When it comes to tube weaning, research has demonstrated that children who consume blended diets experience a number of potential positive outcomes, including:

- Reductions in gagging, retching, and vomiting
- Decreased reflux and dependence on anti-reflux medications
- Normalized stooling and reductions in constipation
- Increased oral intake (Coad et al., 2017)

And when those blended diets are homemade, additional benefits may include:

- Higher parent or caregiver satisfaction
- Lower costs
- Increased involvement in family mealtimes (Novak et al., 2009)

Commercially available blended formulas certainly accomplish the goal of gut priming and challenging the gut. They are also convenient, nutritionally balanced, and easy to use—but they lack variety. Homemade real-food blends provide that variety but are clearly more labor intensive for families. At the same time, parents often report higher levels of satisfaction when they are preparing the foods themselves. The act of feeding is an important part of nurturing, and certainly of parenting, and tube feeding simply does not meet that need in a satisfactory way for many parents. Preparing real-food blends allows parents to share the tastes of their culture with their children, to involve their children in food preparation and cooking, to pass along family traditions, and to satisfy their desire to nurture. Parents often feel empowered and more in control of their child's diet and of their child's health. These are important outcomes that formula feeding often doesn't meet.

With homemade blends, children who are doing some oral feeding can have the very same puree that they eat by mouth fed through their tube. In this way, the smells and tastes (and burps) of the food are the same, whether it went in by mouth or through the tube.

There are some issues to consider, of course. It may go without saying—but let's say it anyway—parents should not embark on a blended diet without the assistance of a registered dietician to help with recipes and strategies that will ensure adequate calories, protein, and vitamins and minerals. Inserting real food through the tube can also clog the tube, but this can often be avoided by using a larger-bore tube (a 14 Fr is generally recommended) and by monitoring the fiber content of the mixtures.

Upon initiation of real-food diets, food allergies or intolerances may become apparent, so parents should be counseled to look for potential allergic signs, including rash or gastric distress or, in severe cases, respiratory distress. As with oral diets, parents should introduce potential allergens one at a time, allowing several days between presentations to monitor for allergic responses. Parents will need appropriate equipment—a heavy-duty blender or food processer—and the ability to prepare and store their blends.

However, not every child (or family) is appropriate for homemade blends. Contraindications include:

- Acute immunosuppression, illness, or medical instability
- G-tube size < 14 Fr
- Infection at the G-tube site
- J-tube (real food *cannot* be used through a J-port)
- Continuous feeding
- Multiple severe food allergies
- Lack of family resources (e.g., electricity, refrigeration, time)

Children who receive tube feedings at school may present additional challenges, as school policies may make it difficult to use homemade real-food blends in some cases. Many schools consider tube feeding a medical procedure that is completed by the school nurse, in the nursing office, under a doctor's order. The variety and lack of standardization of real-food blends may be problematic under these rules. Additionally, schools may lack the ability to refrigerate and store the real-food blends sent from home. In these circumstances, blended diet formulas may be more feasible.

Rapid versus Gradual Weans

How quickly can we reduce calories going through the tube? As quickly as possible, keeping in mind the child's nutritional and medical needs, feeding skills, swallow safety, and family supports. *Rapid weans*, or weans that utilize significant reductions in calories and hunger provocation, are supported by the literature for children who meet certain criteria.

Criteria for rapid weans vary, but all involve a significant reduction in calories provided though the feeding tube. Caloric reductions of 25 to 50 percent have been used successfully to provoke hunger (Kindermann et al., 2008; Krom et al., 2020; Pollow et al., 2018; Wilken et al., 2013). Weight loss is the most common concern voiced by parents and physicians when weaning is being considered. Physicians, in particular, often want to see an increase in calories obtained orally before reducing the calories provided through the tube. However, it is difficult (and perhaps unreasonable) to increase calories by mouth *until* we reduce the calories going through the tube. It is generally agreed in the dietician community that oral nutrition is better utilized by the body. Tube-fed children are often underweight, despite the regular provision of all required (and even higher than required) amounts of nutrients.

Clearly, there are some risks in reducing calories this dramatically, and not all children are good candidates for rapid weans. In most studies, children participating in rapid weans lose weight. Many gain it back once the wean is complete, but this is a risk we need to be aware of and prepare for. Other risks associated with rapid weans include dehydration and nutritional compromise. Careful and regular monitoring of nutrition and hydration status throughout the wean is critical to its success. A plan for rehydration or supplemental tube feeding as needed should be in place. Finally, rapid weans should be time limited. If the child has not transitioned to oral feeding as the primary source of calories within the established time period (generally two to four weeks), the rapid wean should be discontinued.

Your client may be appropriate for a rapid wean if they:

- Are medically and nutritionally stable
- No longer need the tube to manage a medical condition
- Can sustain weight loss

- Have no surgical procedures planned
- Are receiving and tolerating a bolus feeding schedule
- Are receiving feedings on a typical mealtime schedule
- Have oral motor and swallow function that supports oral feeding
- Have a family who is able to commit time and resources to the wean

If the wean is successful, the child will gradually regain any weight loss and begin to gain weight over the next several months. It is not unusual to see periods of food refusal in the months after the wean, particularly if the child is sick or teething.

What about the child who is just not appropriate for a rapid wean? The child who cannot sustain any amount of weight loss or the child who needs to undergo ongoing medical procedures? For these children, we need to consider a more gradual weaning process.

Gradual weans are obviously done more slowly. While a rapid wean is accomplished in several weeks, gradual weans take months to complete. Calories provided through the tube are slowly reduced as oral feeding increases. Tube feeding is reduced by a single bolus, or by 100 to 200 calories at a time in conjunction with increases in oral intake. Establish a mealtime routine with the child, ideally together with family members (or peers at school). Encourage tastes of food during meal and snack times, and as oral intake increases, slowly adjust the calories provided through the tube so the total number of calories remains generally the same. Think of it as a balance scale: As oral calories increase, calories through the tube decrease, maintaining balance throughout the process.

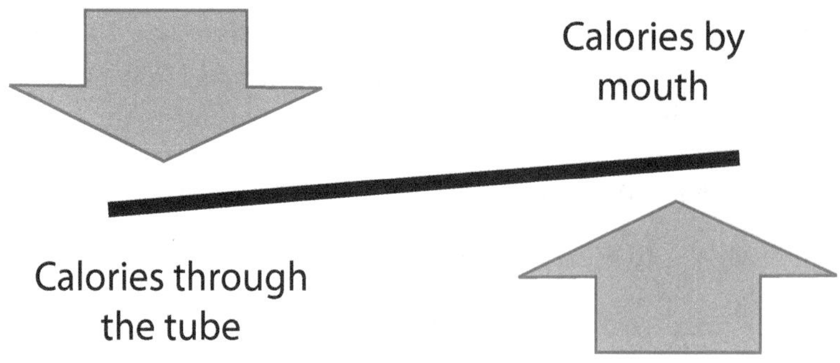

Considerations for Infants

When conducting tube weaning with infants, non-nutritive sucking (typically on a pacifier) can allow the baby to develop sucking skills and reduce the time to transition to full oral feeding. Protocols vary in the literature and in practice. In some protocols, pacifiers are offered before attempts at oral feeding (or before and after), while pacifiers are offered during tube feedings in others. Non-nutritive sucking is associated with a variety of positive outcomes in infants, including (Foster et al., 2016):

- Reduced readiness time for initiation of oral feeding
- Reduced transition time to full oral feeding
- Fewer days in the NICU
- Maintenance of awake, ready state for feeding
- Improved weight gain (in some studies)
- Less oral defensiveness
- More time in calm states
- Better sleep

When working with infants on oral stimulation to prepare them for oral feeding, make sure to use the following protocol:

- Cradle the infant close to your body, as if for feeding. Flexion helps encourage hand-to-mouth coordination.
- Brush the pacifier or your (gloved) finger in a vertical line from the infant's philtrum (i.e., the groove just under the nose), moving down across the lips. An awake, "ready" infant will open their mouth in response. This, in effect, is a request for permission to enter the baby's mouth.
- Once you have permission (i.e., the infant has opened their mouth), place your finger or the pacifier in the baby's mouth. *Never* force your finger or a pacifier into the mouth.
- If the baby does not initiate a suck, provide gentle downward pressure on the tongue.

- Suck stimulation can also be paired with stroking of the facial and oral structures, including the cheeks, lips, gums, and tongue.
- Discontinue any stimulation if the baby becomes irritable or cries.

Infants and children can't always use words to let us know what they need, what they're feeling, or what they want. Learning to watch for their cues, to listen for signs of distress or of comfort, and to pay attention to their responses will make us all more effective feeding therapists.

Appendix I

Sample Feeding and Swallowing Plans

Feeding therapists are often asked to develop home programs, guidelines for school personnel, or programs for early intervention teams to implement. The following pages provide several examples of such plans.

ABC Hospital
Speech-Language Pathology

Patient Name: XX

Date of Birth: 00/00/0000

MRN: 000000

Referring MD: XXX, MD

Date of Report: 00/00/0000

Feeding and Swallowing Guidelines

XX, age 6, participates in speech pathology services at this clinic related to a feeding and swallowing disorder. XX has a diagnosis of chromosomal deletion with resulting hypotonia, developmental delays, and dysphagia. Currently, he presents with a moderate feeding and swallowing disorder characterized by reduced oral motor function, immature mastication, and delays in transition to utensil use. XX is able to use a straw cup independently. He self-feeds finger foods but without external pacing, and he takes very large bites and overfills his mouth, which results in occasional coughing and potential aspiration and choking risk.

XX underwent a modified barium swallow study, which revealed reduced oral control and mild stasis in the cervical esophagus that contribute to reduced food clearance.

The following strategies can be implemented to facilitate XX's intake at school:

1. XX requires supervision at all times with eating. He benefits from verbal prompts to "chew, chew" to promote jaw and tongue movements.
2. XX also requires additional time for eating. XX's chew pattern is immature and is therefore less efficient and takes more time for each bite. He should be given at least 30–35 minutes for lunch to ensure he is able to chew each bite thoroughly and safely. XX does get tired when eating at times and sometimes has difficulty focusing on feeding tasks. He sometimes places his head on the table when eating. Placing a

mirror on the table has been an effective strategy to help him focus on eating, keep his head up, and improve overall feeding efficiency.

3. Pacing is important to XX's safety and to the protection of his airway from aspiration or choking risk. Present small bites of solids (dime to nickel sized), and allow XX time to chew and swallow each bite before giving more. If too much food is placed in front of him, XX will overfill his mouth, which often results in coughing and increased choking risk. Alternating between softer foods and crunchier foods (e.g., a piece of grape, followed by a cracker) also helps XX keep chewing. The softer foods don't always give him enough feedback, and he loses track of where the foods are in his mouth. Following them with something crunchy helps "wake up" his mouth and facilitates more efficient chewing.

4. It is critical to provide upright positioning with sufficient support to ensure XX can maintain an appropriate position with as little effort as possible during feeding activities. XX is better able to protect his airway in this posture and reduce choking risk.

5. Safe and appropriate foods for XX at this time include foods that are cohesive, such as small pieces of sandwiches with soft fillings on toasted bread, cut-up fruit, and dissolvable foods, such as crackers, pretzels, granola, and dry cereal pieces. Avoid foods that are denser (e.g., cake, untoasted bread) and require biting and prolonged chewing. Food that XX's family sends from home will be cut into appropriate sizes for him and be of appropriate texture. Given his food allergies, please avoid giving XX foods that have not been provided by his family.

6. XX can benefit from peer modeling and the socialization that comes with eating with other children, so a transition to eating in the cafeteria will be beneficial for him. Begin with one day per week in order to evaluate his response to the new feeding environment.

7. XX uses a covered straw cup when drinking. If that cup is not available, he can safely drink from a straw placed in an open cup. He will need assistance to hold the cup, to bring it to his mouth, and to maintain placement during drinking.

I am happy to discuss these recommendations in more detail with you. I can be reached at XXX-XXX-XXXX if you have any questions or concerns.

ABC Hospital
Speech-Language Pathology

Patient Name: XX

Date of Birth: 00/00/0000

MRN: 000000

Referring MD: XXX, MD

Date of Report: 00/00/0000

Feeding and Swallowing Guidelines

XX, age 31 months, was referred for speech pathology services related to concerns about feeding and swallowing. She has a diagnosis of periventricular leukomalacia. Evaluation results indicate significant feeding and swallowing deficits characterized by reduced mandibular and lingual function, limited food repertoire, and low volume of intake. Reduced oral motor function results in prolonged mastication, reduced bolus manipulation, and bolus holding. Reduced bolus control appears to result in potential airway compromise, given her intermittent cough noted with eating and drinking during today's evaluation. Given parental report of sensory-seeking behaviors and obvious food refusals, a sensory processing component cannot be ruled out.

Aspiration and choking risk can be reduced by implementing the following strategies:

1. Keep bite sizes small (approximately ¼ inch), and encourage XX to "tuck it in" (i.e., use her tongue to move the food to the side of her mouth to facilitate chewing).

2. When eating with a spoon, use a small, shallow-bowled spoon to help reduce bite size.

Food holding and pocketing can be reduced by implementing the following strategies:

1. Use sips of liquid and/or spoons of pureed food to facilitate clearance of the mouth when pocketing occurs.

2. Routinely alternate between food and liquids to keep pocketing from occurring.

3. Experiment with foods of different temperatures and textures. A crunchy or cold food may help XX resume moving food around in her mouth and assist with clearing the food she is holding.

4. During chewing, encourage XX to chew 2–3 times, then to move the food to the other side of her mouth for 2–3 chews, etc. Moving the food repeatedly across midline may help improve chewing and reduce pocketing.

Activities to improve **oral motor function** include:

1. Place chewy tubing (or similar) at the side of XX's mouth on her teeth. Ask XX to try to use her tongue to move the tubing to the middle of her mouth. Alternately, place the tubing at midline, and ask XX to try to move it to the side of her mouth.

2. Repeat the activity, but include 2–3 repetitions of chewing on the tubing or toy before moving it.

I am happy to discuss these recommendations in more detail with you. I can be reached at XXX-XXX-XXXX if you have any questions or concerns.

ABC Hospital
Speech-Language Pathology

Patient Name: XX

Date of Birth: 00/00/0000

MRN: 000000

Referring MD: XXX, MD

Date of Report: 00/00/0000

Feeding and Swallowing Guidelines

XX is a 14-year-old male child who presents with a moderate to severe feeding disorder characterized by impaired oral mobility and control, limited utensil use, and impaired sensory responses. Repertoire for oral intake is limited to pureed foods, as well as occasional dissolvable solids and thin liquids in small volumes. Swallow function appears to be variable with occasional cough noted. Saliva management has decreased, and drooling is frequent but also varies in severity. Variability in function is likely due to ongoing seizure activity. Nutrition is delivered primarily through a G-tube.

Significant speech and language delays are also present. XX is able to respond to simple yes or no questions with a head shake or nod, although responses are not consistently elicited. Given two food items or utensils, he is able to consistently make a choice to indicate his preference. He is also able to repeat "done, done, done" to indicate his desire for task cessation at times.

XX is seen weekly at this facility for feeding and swallowing therapy with goals of increasing bolus management, increasing volume of oral intake, and improving use of utensils. XX's feeding and swallowing skills are variable.

Aspiration risk can be reduced by implementing the following strategies:

1. Provide upright positioning with sufficient support to ensure XX can maintain an appropriate position with as little effort as possible. Increasing his underlying stability will improve movement in upper extremities for self-feeding, improve pharyngeal swallow response, and increase oral movement for management of foods and liquids.

Appropriate, upright, stable positioning is also important for XX from an energy conservation perspective. That is, energy that XX utilizes to maintain an upright posture is energy that is no longer available to him for safe swallowing. XX's wheelchair provides good positional support for him during feeding tasks.

2. Use small bites and sips as close to midline presentation as possible. This will decrease pocketing and oral residue.

3. Engage in regular oral care to keep XX's mouth as free of bacteria as possible. Aspiration of saliva is not preventable, so it is important to reduce bacteria in the mouth to reduce the risk of aspiration pneumonia. Be sure to clear XX's mouth of any residue after eating.

4. Maintain an upright posture for 20–30 minutes following eating.

The following are suggestions to **improve feeding and swallowing** function:

1. Include XX in the social experience of eating as much as possible. Provide opportunities for participation in classroom lunch and snack activities. Use mealtime language whether XX is eating by mouth or through his tube. For example, use words like *hungry* and *full* during tube feedings.

2. Sensory stimulation prior to feeding is beneficial in alerting or "waking up" XX's muscular and sensory systems. Using intraoral and extraoral vibration, providing XX with a multitextured oral toy, and tapping on his cheeks, chin, and lips can all serve as alerting sensory experiences. This type of stimulation may also be indicated intermittently throughout the meal when oral function appears to decline.

3. Approach XX in a confident manner. Allow him to see the spoon or cup, and talk to him about what is about to happen. XX sometimes becomes defensive during feeding tasks. Don't force foods or utensils into his mouth. Allow him to place the spoon in his mouth, and then guide the spoon to a more midline position to facilitate spoon clearance.

4. Provide breaks if XX appears fatigued or if you hear a wet "gurgly" quality in his vocalizations or exhalations. Sensory stimulation during these breaks can be helpful in improving oral motor movement and re-alerting the muscular system.

I am happy to discuss these recommendations in more detail with you. Please feel free to contact me at XXX-XXX-XXXX if you have any questions or concerns.

ABC Hospital
Speech-Language Pathology

Patient Name: XX

Date of Birth: 00/00/0000

MRN: 000000

Referring MD: XXX, MD

Date of Report: 00/00/0000

Feeding and Swallowing Guidelines

XX is a 30-month-old who was evaluated at this clinic for speech pathology services related to concerns regarding feeding and swallowing. Evaluation revealed significant feeding and swallowing difficulties characterized by over-responsiveness to taste, texture, and novel foods; restrictions in repertoire; and low volume of intake. Mastication with solids (e.g., a raw carrot) was prolonged but was efficient with no post-swallow residue. Swallow response appeared timely with no overt clinical signs or symptoms of aspiration or pharyngeal dysphagia, but liquid trials were limited to a single sip only. Given that XX experiences constipation occasionally, GI discomfort and pressure may be a contributing factor to food refusals.

The following are suggestions for **improving feeding and swallowing** function:

1. Include XX in group snack activities whenever possible. XX will benefit from peer and adult models in regard to food acceptance, utensil use, and other aspect of eating.

2. During meals and snacks, provide XX with preferred foods and at least one new, non-preferred food. Encourage food exploration with the new food (i.e., touching, kissing, licking) without the expectation that she will place it in her mouth initially. Once XX has been able to participate in touching the food item to her face and lips repeatedly, try intraoral placement. Encourage her to "take a bite." Promote self-feeding as much as possible.

3. Include dry spoons, spoons dipped in pureed food, or solid foods in play as much as possible. Touch the utensil or food to her arms, shoulders, cheeks, chin, and lips. Present new foods and liquids in small bites or sips initially so XX does not feel overwhelmed or overstimulated.

4. Always alert XX to what you're doing by using language. For example, before you touch her cheek with the spoon, say "cheek" so she knows what's about to happen. Language will help XX feel more prepared for the feeding activities and can help support sensory processing.

5. Provide XX with verbal praise or access to a preferred toy or activity when she has accomplished interaction with the food or utensil.

I am happy to discuss these recommendations in more detail with you. I can be reached at XXX-XXX-XXXX if you have any questions or concerns.

ABC Hospital
Speech-Language Pathology

Patient Name: XX

Date of Birth: 00/00/0000

MRN: 000000

Referring MD: XXX, MD

Date of Report: 00/00/0000

Feeding and Swallowing Guidelines

XX, age 8, was referred for speech pathology services related to concerns about feeding and swallowing. XX has diagnoses of developmental delays and new onset of epilepsy. XX was accompanied to this evaluation by her parents, who provided all pertinent background information. Medical history is significant for failure to thrive, esophagitis, eosinophilic esophagitis, gastroesophageal reflux disease, and attention-deficit/hyperactivity disorder. In addition, she was hospitalized twice in a six-month period with aspiration pneumonia, and a modified barium swallow study completed at XX Children's Hospital revealed aspiration with thin liquids. An endoscopic study with otolaryngology confirmed these results. A diet of soft solids and liquids thickened to "half nectar" was recommended.

Evaluation at this clinic revealed a moderate feeding and swallowing disorder characterized by slowed bolus management and propulsion, immature mastication pattern, and known pharyngeal dysphagia per the previous swallow study. Oral motor function is significant for reduced tone, slowed lingual and jaw movements, lack of rotary jaw movement with chew, and incomplete lip, tongue, and jaw differentiation. Labial closure is achieved intermittently, and occasional anterior bolus loss is noted.

Aspiration and choking risk can be reduced by implementing the following strategies:

1. **Seating:** Be sure XX is in supported seating, including upright posture, base of support for her feet, and lateral supports for postural stability. A chair that allows XX to reach the table and maintain eye contact with

the feeder will facilitate appropriate pace and supervision, as well as self-feeding as possible.

2. **Diet:** Continue with diet as recommended following the modified barium swallow study, specifically soft solids and "half nectar" liquids. Provide soft solids in small bites and pieces. Utilize a slowed rate to ensure XX has cleared her mouth before each bite. Limit harder-to-manage foods to home mealtimes or to therapeutic trials to maximize caloric input during school mealtimes.
3. **Supervision/assistance:** XX requires assistance from a feeder. Encourage her to participate in self-feeding as possible. Limit mealtimes to 30–45 minutes to maximize metabolism and avoid burning more calories than XX takes in.

Mastication (chewing) and oral management can be maximized by implementing the following strategies:

1. **Food placement:** Place foods that require chewing on the sides of XX's mouth whenever possible. This will facilitate vertical jaw movements and lateral tongue movements.
2. **Food types:** Foods with natural cohesion (i.e., those that "stick together") will facilitate improved oral management and reduce food loss. Examples include foods that are soft, moist, and easily formed into a bolus, including ground meats with gravies, soft cooked pasta, and soft cooked vegetables.

Therapeutic exercises and activities to improve **oral motor function** include:

1. Place chewy tubing (or similar) at the side of XX's mouth on her teeth. Ask XX to try to use her tongue to move the tubing to the middle of her mouth. Alternately, place the tubing at midline, and ask XX to try to move it to the side of her mouth. This can also be accomplished with food items, such as lollipops, licorice sticks, and cheese sticks.
2. Repeat the activity, but include 2–3 repetitions of chewing on the tubing or toy before moving it.

I am happy to discuss these recommendations in more detail with you. I can be reached at XXX-XXX-XXXX if you have any questions or concerns.

Appendix II
Goal Writing Suggestions

All treatment goals need to meet three standards: They have to be *measurable*, *observable*, and *objective*. Concepts like "improved chew" or "safe intake" are not quantifiable or observable. Ask yourself: Can I measure this? How will I know my client has reached this goal? You can choose from a variety of potential criterion to help you define your goal, depending on the client, the task, and the intervention area:

- Percent accurate (e.g., "with 90 percent accuracy")
- Time period (e.g., "for 2 minutes")
- Minimum number of responses (e.g., "5–8 times per meal")
- Maximum number of errors (e.g., "with no more than 3 episodes of bolus loss")
- Number of cues (e.g., "with no more than 3 prompts from feeder")

When writing goals for feeding and swallowing skills, think about what you want to accomplish, rather than the tools you're using to get there. Writing a goal for chewing on a chewy tube or for blowing cotton balls across a table doesn't tell the reviewer *why* you are doing that activity. Instead, write a goal for rotary mastication or improved respiratory-swallow coordination. The focus is on function: What is the functional eating goal that these activities are helping the client work toward? The following table provides some examples of short- and long-term goals in a variety of intervention areas. They are not presented in a hierarchy but are designed to provide a number of different examples so you can choose the goal and criterion that works for you, your client, and your setting.

Intervention	Short-Term Goals	Long-Term Goals
Expanding repertoire	• Client will participate in food exploration of novel foods with minimal cueing from the clinician/caregiver • Client will accept, chew, and swallow small bites of novel foods 20–30 times per session • Client will expand their food repertoire to include 2–3 novel foods	• Client will utilize food exploration strategies at an independent level • Client will expand their food repertoire to include 6–8 novel foods
Improving chew/bite	• Client will demonstrate bolus lateralization with solid boluses 5–8 times per session • Client will demonstrate repeated vertical jaw movements with dissolvable solids in 50 percent of trials • Client will demonstrate rotary jaw movements during mastication of solid foods 10–15 times per session or meal	• Client will manage solid boluses at an independent level • Client will demonstrate independent management of soft solid foods
Utensil use (spoon)	• Client will demonstrate labial closure and clearance of puree from a shallow spoon in 90 percent of trials • Client will demonstrate labial closure and clearance of thick puree from a spoon 5–8 times per session • Client will use lips to clear boluses from a spoon 10–12 times per session	• Client will eat soft solid foods from a spoon at an independent level • Client will clear puree and soft boluses from a spoon in 90 percent of trials

Intervention	Short-Term Goals	Long-Term Goals
Utensil use (cup)	• Client will demonstrate labial closure with cup sips in 90 percent of trials • Client will demonstrate an ability to sip from a small open cup 20–25 times per session or meal • Client will sip from a covered cup with no more than 3 episodes of bolus loss per meal	• Client will demonstrate independent use of a covered cup with a straw • Client will demonstrate independent management of liquids via an open cup in 90 percent of trials
Utensil use (straw)	• Client will demonstrate labial closure with a straw 5–8 times per session • Client will draw liquid through a straw 6–8 times per session • Client will sip liquid via a straw with no more than 2 episodes of bolus loss	• Client will demonstrate independent use of straw in 90 percent of trials
Breathing-swallow coordination	• Client will demonstrate post-swallow exhalation in 50 percent of liquid trials • Client will utilize a slower rate of intake with no more than 3 prompts from the feeder • Client will demonstrate dyspnea during drinking tasks no more than 8 times per meal	• Client will demonstrate post-swallow exhalation in 90 percent of trials • Client will demonstrate dyspnea during drinking tasks no more than 2 times per meal

Appendix III

Teletherapy Tips

When I began writing this book (and, in fact, for most of my career), my therapy sessions were taking place in hospital rooms, our clinic, or my client's classroom, cafeteria, or home. In March of 2020, my life—like all of yours—changed dramatically. The COVID-19 pandemic closed our clinic for two months, and when we resumed outpatient services, we did so exclusively via telehealth. Even when the clinic began to open to clients, many of my clients, particularly the more fragile and medically complex, chose to continue virtual visits to protect their health. It has been quite a learning experience for this old therapist, and it occurred to me that it might be useful to share some of the things I've learned about feeding and swallowing therapy via telehealth.

Communicating via Videoconference

- **Slow down:** Speaking at a slightly slower rate gives your client additional time to process the information you're providing. A slower rate also helps in the event there is mis-synchrony between audio and video feeds.
- **Articulate clearly:** Precise articulation is always important to communication, but it's particularly important when audio connections may not be as clear as we'd like.
- **Maintain eye contact:** It's easy to get distracted when communicating via video or teleconference, but when you're on screen, be sure to look at the camera and not away at whatever else might be going on in your environment. When others are on screen, maintain eye contact with them as much as possible too.
- **Use prosody and intonation:** Voice is an important tool in communication and in therapy and can help keep the child's attention on you. Be sure to keep your voice animated. Remember, prosody communicates a great deal of meaning. Think about the difference

between a *hot* dog (which you might want for lunch) and a hot *dog* (which you definitely wouldn't want to eat!). The difference is emphasis, and we can use prosodic emphasis to convey meaning and call our listener's attention to whatever aspect of our message we want to highlight.

- **Minimize distractions:** Easy to say but hard to do, right? To the extent that you can, reduce the potential distractors around you so your communication partner (or partners) can focus on you and your message. Find a quiet place to do your teleconferencing so background noise is at a minimum.

- **Simplify your message***:* Resist the urge to use long explanations and descriptions. Be direct, and provide as much redundancy in your message as you can. Use additional visual cues or materials whenever possible to enhance your message.

Pre-Session Prep

In some ways, feeding and swallowing therapy treatments are uniquely suited for telehealth since home is where our clients eat most of the time. We can get a good look at the child's typical feeding environment, evaluate their seating and positioning in their kitchen or dining room, and meet all of their mealtime partners (including dogs and cats!)—all via our computer screens. Some preparation before the session will make things go more smoothly:

- **Location, location:** Talk with the child's parents or caregivers ahead of time about where the session will take place. Do you want the child in a particular seat? At a table? Positioned in a particular way? Perhaps you want to be able to see where the child typically eats.

- **Plan the menu:** Spend a few minutes (via phone, videochat, or email) with the parents or caregivers planning for the visit. They will need to have food and utensils ready to go, so decide together what you'll be working on before the session begins. I typically ask them to have one or two "easy" foods and one or two "new" foods available.

- **It's still okay to play:** Have other activities available the same way you would during an in-person session. You can incorporate online games and e-books into your feeding activities by screen-sharing. Some of my clients and I draw pictures together on the Zoom whiteboard. Others prefer reading stories via the e-reader app. Most of the activities you incorporate into your in-person sessions can be digitally adapted. Just be sure to have them open on your computer ahead of time so you can access them easily once your televisit gets going.

During the Session

- **Ready for your close-up?** Position the camera so the child can easily see your face and any mouth movements you make. Ask the grown-ups on the other end to position their camera so you can see the child's face and mouth clearly.
- **We're all still eating together:** The same rule applies—everybody eats! If you've planned which foods you're working on ahead of time, you can have something similar available to eat yourself. Model food exploration, biting, and chewing in the same way you would if you were all in the same room, sitting at the same table. Even if what you're eating is different from what the child is eating, you're eating together.
- **Collaborate:** It is often a logistical nightmare to get parents, dieticians, therapists, applied behavior analysis clinicians, and so on in a single room at the same time for collaboration. Virtual sessions give us the unique opportunity to include a variety of team members in a single session, so take advantage and invite other team members to your visits.
- **Frame your face:** When demonstrating or modeling, keep the child's attention on your face. Hold the food or utensil high, next to or in front of your face to be sure it is "in the frame" and that your client can see you and it clearly. Foods or utensils that are on a plate or on the table in front of you will not be visible to the child in the way they would be if you were sitting together at the same table.
- **Be flexible:** Things won't always go as planned—connections can be lost and children can wander away from the screen—but this really isn't any different than in-person sessions, is it? Have a backup plan, and be prepared to work with the parents to troubleshoot together.
- **Keep the finishing details in mind:** As the session ends, provide the parents with feedback about feeding and swallowing skills *and* about issues related to the virtual format. Decide together what worked and what didn't, and make a plan for subsequent sessions.

And finally, relax! You know how to conduct a therapy session and have been doing it successfully for a long time, haven't you? Yes, you may be using new tools, but therapy is still therapy.

Glossary

Airway: Passages through which air travels during respiration

Alveoli: Small spaces along the walls of the alveolar sacs; the majority of the gas exchange in respiration occurs in the alveoli and alveolar sacs

Apnea: Breathing cessation

Arytenoid cartilages: Pair of pyramid-shped cartilages that are part of the larynx; important in vocal fold movement; contact the underside of the epiglottis during swallowing to seal the airway

Aspiration: Foreign material (e.g., food, liquid, secretions, refluxate) that enters the airway and moves through the vocal folds into the trachea

Bilevel positive airway pressure (BiPAP): A device that provides ventilation without need for intubation

Bolus: A mass of food or liquid to be swallowed

Bronchi: Large air passages in the lungs

Bronchiectasis: Abnormal widening of the bronchial tubes, typically with infection

Bronchioles: Small air passages in the lungs

Bronchiolitis: Inflammation of the bronchioles

Bronchitis: Inflammation of the bronchi

Bruxism: Grinding of teeth

Chemesthesis: Sensations activated by chemical compounds, such as the burn from hot peppers or the sting of carbonation

Cilia: Hair-like structures that line the bronchi and bronchioles; move in waves in the lung fluid

Dysphagia: Disordered swallowing

Endotracheal tube: Tube inserted into the trachea to maintain an open airway and to connect to a ventilator

Epiglottis: Leaf-shaped cartilage attached to the tongue base; inverts to cover the airway during swallowing

Esophagus: Muscular tube that connects the pharynx to the stomach

Flexion: Bending

Frenulum: Membrane underneath the oral tongue

Hard palate: Bony portion of the roof of the mouth

High-flow nasal cannula (HFNC): Oxygen delivery via a specialized cannula that allows for flow rate of 40–60 lpm

Hyoid bone: U-shaped bone at the base of tongue; point of attachment for tongue muscles superiorly and muscles responsible for laryngeal elevation inferiorly

Hyolaryngeal complex: The hyoid bone and larynx, functioning as a unit to close the airway during swallowing

Interoception: Perception of internal sensation

Laryngospasm: Spasm of the larynx; results in breathing cessation

Larynx: Portion of the airway between the pharynx and the trachea; houses the vocal folds

Macronutrients: Nutrients required in large amounts by the body, including fats, proteins, and carbohydrates
Mandible: Lower portion of the jaw
Mastication: Chewing
Mechanical ventilation: The use of mechanical means, typically a ventilator, to replace or assist with spontaneous breathing
Microbiome: The collection of microorganisms that occupy a particular area, such as the gut or the skin
Micronutrients: Nutrients required in small amounts by the body, including vitamins and minerals
Motor unit: A motor neuron and the muscle fibers it controls
Nasal airway: Portion of the upper respiratory tract that includes the nasal passages
Neuroplasticity: Brain changes that occur in response to activity or experience
Noninvasive positive pressure ventilation (NPPV): Mechanical ventilation provided via a mask or nasal cannula rather than an endotracheal tube
Non-nutritive sucking: Sucking without feeding (e.g., on a pacifier)
Nutritive sucking: Sucking for feeding (e.g., on a bottle or the breast)
Oral: Pertaining to the mouth
Paradoxical vocal fold movement (PVFM): A voice disorder in which the vocal folds close when they should be opening
Penetration: Foreign matter (e.g., food, liquids, reflux) that enters the airway but does not proceed past the vocal folds
Phagocytosis: Process by which cells ingest microorganisms and foreign particles
Pharynx: The throat
Phasic bite reflex: Reflexive opening and closing of the jaw; triggered by stimulation to the gums
Pneumonia: Infection of the lungs
Pulmonary: Relating to the lungs and lung function
Pulmonary clearance: Removal of foreign material from the airways
Reflux: Backflow of stomach contents into the esophagus or pharynx
Respiration: The exchange of oxygen and carbon dioxide between the atmosphere and the cells of the body
Rooting reflex: Reflexive turning of the head in infants; triggered by touch to the cheek or lips
Soft palate: The soft, muscular portion of the palate; the posterior portion of the roof of the mouth
Stridor: Noisy breathing, typically as a result of airway obstruction
Suckling pads: Fat pads in the cheeks of infants that provide stability during sucking and help to direct the bolus through the oral cavity
Surfactant: Foamy fluid in the lungs that keeps alveoli open and available for gas exchange
Trachea: The portion of the airway between the larynx and the bronchi of the lungs

Tracheostomy: Surgical insertion in the trachea through which a tube is inserted for attachment to mechanical ventilation or to provide access to the lungs for suctioning

Transverse tongue reflex: Reflexive lateralization of the tongue; triggered by touch to the side of the tongue

Vallecula: The spaces between the base of the tongue and the epiglottis, right and left

Velum: The soft palate

Ventilation: The mechanical movement of air through the respiratory system

Vocal folds: Folds of tissue in the larynx that adduct for voice production and close the airway during swallowing (also known as vocal cords)

Vocal tract: Cavities where sound is produced and modified, including the larynx, pharynx, and oral and nasal cavities

Waterbrash: Excessive salivation triggered by excessive reflux (also known as esophago-salivary reflex)

Work of breathing: The energy required to move air through the airways and to expand the lungs against the natural recoil of the ribcage

References

For your convenience, purchasers can download and print worksheets and handouts from www.pesi.com/Mansolillo

American Psychiatric Association. (2013). *Diagnostic and statistical manual of mental disorders* (5th ed.). https://doi.org/10.1176/appi.books.9780890425596

American Speech-Language-Hearing Association. (2019). *SLP health care survey report: Caseload characteristics, 2005–2019.* https://www.asha.org/siteassets/surveys/2019-slp-health-care-survey-caseload-characteristics-and-trends-2005-2019.pdf

American Speech-Language-Hearing Association. (2020). *Schools survey report: SLP caseload characteristics trends, 2004–2020.* https://www.asha.org/siteassets/surveys/2020-schools-survey-caseload-characteristics-trends.pdf

Arvedson, J., Brodsky, L., & Lefton-Greif, M. (2020). *Pediatric swallowing and feeding assessment and management* (3rd ed.). Plural Publishing.

Bahia, M. M., & Lowell, S. Y. (2020). A systematic review of the physiological effects of the effortful swallow maneuver in adults with normal and disordered swallowing. *American Journal of Speech-Language Pathology, 29*(3), 1–19.

Beall, M. H., van den Wijngaard, J. P., van Gemert, M. J., & Ross, M. G. (2007). Regulation of amniotic fluid volume. *Placenta, 28*(8–9), 824–832.

Britton, D., Hoit, J. D., Benditt, J. O., Poon, J., Hansen, M., Baylor, C. R., & Yorkston, K. M. (2020). Swallowing with noninvasive positive-pressure ventilation (NPPV) in individuals with muscular dystrophy: A qualitative analysis. *Dysphagia, 35*(1), 32–41.

Caldwell, A. R., Terhorst, L., Skidmore, E. R., & Bendixen, R. M. (2018). Is frequency of family meals associated with fruit and vegetable intake among preschoolers? A logistic regression analysis. *Journal of Human Nutrition and Dietetics, 31*(4), 505–512.

Carlaw, C., Finlayson, H., Beggs, K., Visser, T., Marcoux, C., Coney, D., & Steele, C. M. (2012). Outcomes of a pilot water protocol project in a rehabilitation setting. *Dysphagia, 27*(3), 297–306.

Case-Smith, J., Weaver, L. L., & Fristad, M. A. (2015). A systematic review of sensory processing interventions for children with autism spectrum disorders. *Autism, 19*(2), 133–148.

Cerny, F. J., Panzarella, K. J., & Stathopoulos, E. (1997). Expiratory muscle conditioning in hypotonic children with low vocal intensity levels. *Journal of Medical Speech-Language Pathology, 5*(2), 141–152.

Ceunen, E., Vlaeyen, J. W., & van Diest, I. (2016). On the origin of interoception. *Frontiers in Psychology, 7*, Article 743.

Chang, Y. J., Lin, C. P., Lin, Y. J., & Lin, C. H. (2007). Effects of single-hole and cross-cut nipple units on feeding efficiency and physiological parameters in premature infants. *The Journal of Nursing Research, 15*(3), 215–223.

Cichero, J. A. (2013). Thickening agents used for dysphagia management: Effect on bioavailability of water, medication and feelings of satiety. *Nutrition Journal, 12*(1), 1–8.

Clarke, G., O'Mahony, S. M., Dinan, T. G., & Cryan, J. F. (2014). Priming for health: Gut microbiota acquired in early life regulates physiology, brain and behaviour. *Acta Paediatrica, 103*(8), 812–819.

Coad, J., Toft, A., Lapwood, S., Manning, J., Hunter, M., Jenkins, H., & Widdas, D. (2017). Blended foods for tube-fed children: A safe and realistic option? A rapid review of the evidence. *Archives of Disease in Childhood, 102,* 274–278.

Cole, N. C., Musaad, S. M., Lee, S. Y., Donovan, S. M., & The STRONG Kids Team. (2018). Home feeding environment and picky eating behavior in preschool-aged children: A prospective analysis. *Eating Behaviors, 30,* 76–82.

Craig, A. D. (2002). How do you feel? Interoception: The sense of the physiological condition of the body. *Nature Reviews Neuroscience, 3*(8), 655–666.

Curtis, J. A., & Troche, M. S. (2020). Effects of verbal cueing on respiratory-swallow patterning, lung volume initiation, and swallow apnea duration in Parkinson's disease. *Dysphagia, 35*(3), 460–470.

Daniels, S. K., & Foundas, A. L. (2001). Swallowing physiology of sequential straw drinking. *Dysphagia, 16*(3), 176–182.

DeGrace, B. W., Foust, R. E., Sisson, S. B., & Lora, K. R. (2016). Benefits of family meals for children with special therapeutic and behavioral needs. *American Journal of Occupational Therapy, 70*(3), Article 7003350010.

Douglas, P., & Geddes, D. (2018). Practice-based interpretation of ultrasound studies leads the way to more effective clinical support and less pharmaceutical and surgical intervention for breastfeeding infants. *Midwifery, 58,* 145–155.

Dozier, T. S., Brodsky, M. B., Michel, Y., Walters Jr., B. C., & Martin-Harris, B. (2006). Coordination of swallowing and respiration in normal sequential cup swallows. *The Laryngoscope, 116*(8), 1489–1493.

Dunlop, A. L., Mulle, J. G., Ferranti, E. P., Edwards, S., Dunn, A. B., & Corwin, E. J. (2015). The maternal microbiome and pregnancy outcomes that impact infant health: A review. *Advances in Neonatal Care, 15*(6), 377–385.

Ferrara, L., Kamity, R., Islam, S., Sher, I., Barlev, D., Wennerholm, L., Redstone, F., & Hanna, N. (2018). Short-term effects of cold liquids on the pharyngeal swallow in preterm infants with dysphagia: A pilot study. *Dysphagia, 33*(5), 593–601.

Forestell, C. A. (2017). Flavor perception and preference development in human infants. *Annals of Nutrition and Metabolism, 70*(Suppl. 3), 17–25.

Foster, J. P., Psaila, K., & Patterson, T. (2016). Non-nutritive sucking for increasing physiologic stability and nutrition in preterm infants. *Cochrane Database of Systematic Reviews.* https://doi.org/10.1002/14651858.CD001071.pub3

Frazier, J. B., & Friedman, B. (1996). Swallow function in children with Down syndrome: A retrospective study. *Developmental Medicine & Child Neurology, 38*(8), 695–703.

Frey, K. L., & Ramsberger, G. (2011). Comparison of outcomes before and after implementation of a water protocol for patients with cerebrovascular accident and dysphagia. *Journal of Neuroscience Nursing, 43*(3), 165–171.

Fucile, S., McFarland, D. H., Gisel, E. G., & Lau, C. (2012). Oral and nonoral sensorimotor interventions facilitate suck-swallow-respiration functions and their coordination in preterm infants. *Early Human Development, 88*(6), 345–350.

Gillman, A., Winkler, R., & Taylor, N. F. (2017). Implementing the free water protocol does not result in aspiration pneumonia in carefully selected patients with dysphagia: A systematic review. *Dysphagia, 32*(3), 345–361.

Goday, P. S., Huh, S. Y., Silverman, A., Lukens, C. T., Dodrill, P., Cohen, S. S., Delaney, A. L., Feuling, M. B., Noel, R. J., Gisel, E., Kenzer, A., Kessler, D. B., Kraus de Camargo, O., Browne, J., & Phalen, J. A. (2019). Pediatric feeding disorder: Consensus definition and conceptual framework. *Journal of Pediatric Gastroenterology and Nutrition, 68*(1), 124–129.

Goldberg, E., Barton, S., Xanthopoulos, M. S., Stettler, N., & Liacouras, C. A. (2010). A descriptive study of complications of gastrostomy tubes in children. *Journal of Pediatric Nursing, 25*(2), 72–80.

Goldin, A. B., Heiss, K. F., Hall, M., Rothstein, D. H., Minneci, P. C., Blakely, M. L., Browne, M., Raval, M. V., Shah, S. S., Rangel, S. J., Snyder, C. L., Vinocur, C. D., Berman, L., Cooper, J. N., & Arca, M. J. (2016). Emergency department visits and readmissions among children after gastrostomy tube placement. *The Journal of Pediatrics, 174*, 139–145.

Griffin, S. O., Wei, L., Gooch, B. F., Weno, K., & Espinoza, L. (2016). Vital signs: Dental sealant use and untreated tooth decay among US school-aged children. *Morbidity and Mortality Weekly Report, 65*(41), 1141–1145.

Hirsch, A. W., Monuteaux, M. C., Fruchtman, G., Bachur, R. G., & Neuman, M. I. (2016). Characteristics of children hospitalized with aspiration pneumonia. *Hospital Pediatrics, 6*(11), 659–666.

Hirst, K., Dodrill, P., & Gosa, M. (2017). Noninvasive respiratory support and feeding in the neonate. *Perspectives of the ASHA Special Interest Groups, 2*(13), 82–92.

Hiss, S. G., Treole, K., & Stuart, A. (2001). Effects of age, gender, bolus volume, and trial on swallowing apnea duration and swallow/respiratory phase relationships of normal adults. *Dysphagia, 16*(2), 128–135.

Hoffmeister, J., Zaborek, N., & Thibeault, S. L. (2019). Postextubation dysphagia in pediatric populations: Incidence, risk factors, and outcomes. *The Journal of Pediatrics, 211*, 126–133.

Indrio, F., Riezzo, G., Tafuri, S., Ficarella, M., Carlucci, B., Bisceglia, M., Polimeno, L., & Francavilla, R. (2017). Probiotic supplementation in preterm: Feeding intolerance and hospital cost. *Nutrients, 9*(9), Article 965.

Jackson, K. D., Howie, L. D., & Akinbami, L. J. (2013). *Trends in allergic conditions among children: United States, 1997–2011* (NCHS Data Brief No. 121). US Department of Health and Human Services, Centers for Disease Control and Prevention, National Center for Health Statistics.

Karagiannis, M. J., Chivers, L., & Karagiannis, T. C. (2011). Effects of oral intake of water in patients with oropharyngeal dysphagia. *BMC Geriatrics, 11*(1), Article 9.

Karagiannis, M., & Karagiannis, T. C. (2014). Oropharyngeal dysphagia, free water protocol and quality of life: An update from a prospective clinical trial. *Hellenic Journal of Nuclear Medicine, 17*(1), 26–29.

Kennedi, H., Campbell-Vance, J., Reynolds, J., Foreman, M., Dollaghan, C., Graybeal, D., Warren, A. M., & Bennett, M. (2019). Implementation and analysis of a free water protocol in acute trauma and stroke patients. *Critical Care Nurse, 39*(3), e9–e17.

Khoshoo, V., & Edell, D. (1999). Previously healthy infants may have increased risk of aspiration during respiratory syncytial viral bronchiolitis. *Pediatrics, 104*(6), 1389–1390.

Kindermann, A., Kneepkens, C. M. F., Stok, A., van Dijk, E. M., Engels, M., & Douwes, A. C. (2008). Discontinuation of tube feeding in young children by hunger provocation. *Journal of Pediatric Gastroenterology and Nutrition, 47*(1), 87–91.

Krom, H., de Meij, T. G., Benninga, M. A., van Dijk-Lokkart, E. M., Engels, M., Kneepkens, C. F., Kuiper-Cramer, L., Otten, M. G. M., van der Sluijs Veer, L., Stok-Akerboom, A. M., Zilverberg, R., van Zundert, S. M. C., & Kindermann, A. (2020). Long-term efficacy of clinical hunger provocation to wean feeding tube dependent children. *Clinical Nutrition, 39*(9), 2863–2871.

Krom, H., de Winter, J. P., & Kindermann, A. (2017). Development, prevention, and treatment of feeding tube dependency. *European Journal of Pediatrics, 176*(6), 683–688.

Lau, C. (2016). Development of infant oral feeding skills: What do we know? *The American Journal of Clinical Nutrition, 103*(2), 616S–621S.

Lee, S. Y., Ha, S. A., Seo, J. S., Sohn, C. M., Park, H. R., & Kim, K. W. (2014). Eating habits and eating behaviors by family dinner frequency in the lower-grade elementary school students. *Nutrition Research and Practice, 8*(6), 679–687.

Lundine, J. P., Bates, D. G., & Yin, H. (2015). Analysis of carbonated thin liquids in pediatric neurogenic dysphagia. *Pediatric Radiology, 45*(9), 1323–1332.

Martin-Harris, B., McFarland, D., Hill, E. G., Strange, C. B., Focht, K. L., Wan, Z., Blair, J., & McGrattan, K. (2015). Respiratory-swallow training in patients with head and neck cancer. *Archives of Physical Medicine and Rehabilitation, 96*(5), 885–893.

Massery, M. (1991). Chest development as a component of normal motor development: Implications for pediatric physical therapists. *Pediatric Physical Therapy, 3*(1), 3–8.

McSweeney, M. E., Kerr, J., Jiang, H., & Lightdale, J. R. (2015). Risk factors for complications in infants and children with percutaneous endoscopic gastrostomy tubes. *The Journal of Pediatrics, 166*(6), 1514–1519.

Mennella, J. A. (1995). Mother's milk: A medium for early flavor experiences. *Journal of Human Lactation, 11*(1), 39–45.

Mennella, J. A., Jagnow, C. P., & Beauchamp, G. K. (2001). Prenatal and postnatal flavor learning by human infants. *Pediatrics, 107*(6), e88–e88.

Mikalsen, I. B., Davis, P., & Øymar, K. (2016). High flow nasal cannula in children: A literature review. *Scandinavian Journal of Trauma, Resuscitation and Emergency Medicine, 24*, Article 93.

Milani, C., Duranti, S., Bottacini, F., Casey, E., Turroni, F., Mahony, J., Belzer, C., Delgado Palacio, S., Arboleya Montes, S., Mancabelli, L., Lugli, G. A., Rodriguez, J. M., Bode, L., de Vos, W., Gueimonde, M., Margolles, A., van Sinderen, D., & Ventura, M. (2017). The first microbial colonizers of the human gut: Composition, activities, and health implications of the infant gut microbiota. *Microbiology and Molecular Biology Reviews, 81*(4), Article e00036-17.

Miller, J. L., Sonies, B. C., & Macedonia, C. (2003). Emergence of oropharyngeal, laryngeal and swallowing activity in the developing fetal upper aerodigestive tract: An ultrasound evaluation. *Early Human Development, 71*(1), 61–87.

Mills, N., Pransky, S. M., Geddes, D. T., & Mirjalili, S. A. (2019). What is a tongue tie? Defining the anatomy of the in-situ lingual frenulum. *Clinical Anatomy, 32*(6), 749–761.

Mills, R. H., & Ashford, J. R. (2008). A methodology for the inclusion of laboratory assessment in the evaluation of dysphagia. *Perspectives on Swallowing and Swallowing Disorders (Dysphagia), 17*(4), 128–134.

Murray, J., Doeltgen, S., Miller, M., & Scholten, I. (2016). Does a water protocol improve the hydration and health status of individuals with thin liquid aspiration following stroke? A randomized controlled trial. *Dysphagia, 31*(3), 424–433.

Nadon, G., Feldman, D. E., Dunn, W., & Gisel, E. (2011). Association of sensory processing and eating problems in children with autism spectrum disorders. *Autism Research and Treatment, 2011*, Article 541926.

Nagy, A., Leigh, C., Hori, S. F., Molfenter, S. M., Shariff, T., & Steele, C. M. (2013). Timing differences between cued and noncued swallows in healthy young adults. *Dysphagia, 28*(3), 428–434.

Newman, R., Vilardell, N., Clavé, P., & Speyer, R. (2016). Effect of bolus viscosity on the safety and efficacy of swallowing and the kinematics of the swallow response in patients with oropharyngeal dysphagia: White paper by the European Society for Swallowing Disorders (ESSD). *Dysphagia, 31*(2), 232–249.

Novak, P., Wilson, K. E., Ausderau, K., & Cullinane, D. (2009). The use of blenderized tube feedings. *ICAN: Infant, Child, & Adolescent Nutrition, 1*(1), 21–23.

O'Shea, J. E., Foster, J. P., O'Donnell, C. P., Breathnach, D., Jacobs, S. E., Todd, D. A., & Davis, P. G. (2017). Frenotomy for tongue-tie in newborn infants. *Cochrane Database of Systematic Reviews.* https://doi.org/10.1002/14651858.CD011065.pub2

Panther, K. (2005). The Frazier free water protocol. *Perspectives on Swallowing and Swallowing Disorders (Dysphagia), 14*(1), 4–9.

Payne, C., Methven, L., Fairfield, C., & Bell, A. (2011). Consistently inconsistent: Commercially available starch-based dysphagia products. *Dysphagia, 26*(1), 27–33.

Pinnington, L. L., Smith, C. M., Ellis, R. E., & Morton, R. E. (2000). Feeding efficiency and respiratory integration in infants with acute viral bronchiolitis. *The Journal of Pediatrics, 137*(4), 523–526.

Pollow, A. S., Karls, C. A., Witzlib, M., Noel, R. J., Goday, P. S., & Silverman, A. H. (2018). Safety of appetite manipulation in children with feeding disorders admitted to an inpatient feeding program. *Journal of Pediatric Gastroenterology and Nutrition, 66*(5), e127–e130.

Pooyania, S., Vandurme, L., Daun, R., & Buchel, C. (2015). Effects of a free water protocol on inpatients in a neuro-rehabilitation setting. *Open Journal of Therapy and Rehabilitation, 3*(4), 132–138.

Rosen, R., Vandenplas, Y., Singendonk, M., Cabana, M., DiLorenzo, C., Gottrand, F., Gupta, S., Langendam, M., Staiano, A., Thapar, N., Tipnis, N., & Tabbers, M. (2018). Pediatric gastroesophageal reflux clinical practice guidelines: Joint recommendations of the North American Society for Pediatric Gastroenterology, Hepatology, and Nutrition and the European Society for Pediatric Gastroenterology, Hepatology, and Nutrition. *Journal of Pediatric Gastroenterology and Nutrition, 66*(3), 516–554.

Schwarz, S. M. (2003). Feeding disorders in children with developmental disabilities. *Infants & Young Children, 16*(4), 317–330.

Schwarz, S. M., Corredor, J., Fisher-Medina, J., Cohen, J., & Rabinowitz, S. (2001). Diagnosis and treatment of feeding disorders in children with developmental disabilities. *Pediatrics, 108*(3), 67–676.

Shekerdemian, L. S., Mahmood, N. R., Wolfe, K. K., Riggs, B. J., Ross, C. E., McKiernan, C. A., Heidemann, S. M., Kleinman, L. C., Sen, A. I., Hall, M. W., Priestley, M. A., McGuire, J. K., Boukas, K., Sharron, M. P., & Burns, J. P. (2020). Characteristics and outcomes of children with coronavirus disease 2019 (COVID-19) infection admitted to US and Canadian pediatric intensive care units. *JAMA Pediatrics, 174*(9), 868–873.

Sia, I., Crary, M. A., Kairalla, J., Carnaby, G. D., Sheplak, M., & McCulloch, T. (2018). Bolus volume and viscosity effects on pharyngeal swallowing power—How physiological bolus accommodation affects bolus dynamics. *Neurogastroenterology & Motility, 30*(12), Article e13481.

Steele, C. M., Namasivayam-MacDonald, A. M., Guida, B. T., Cichero, J. A., Duivestein, J., Hanson, B., Lam, P., & Riquelme, L. F. (2018). Creation and initial validation of the international dysphagia diet standardisation initiative functional diet scale. *Archives of Physical Medicine and Rehabilitation, 99*(5), 934–944.

Stewart, C. J., Ajami, N. J., O'Brien, J. L., Hutchinson, D. S., Smith, D. P., Wong, M. C., Ross, M. C., Llyod, R. E., Doddapaneni, H., Metcalf, G. A., Muzny, D., Gibbs, R. A., Vatanen, T., Huttenhower, C., Xavier, R. J., Rewers, M., Hagopian, W., Toppari, J., Ziegler, A-G., ... Petrosino, J. F. (2018). Temporal development of the gut microbiome in early childhood from the TEDDY study. *Nature, 562*(7728), 583–588.

Suskind, D. L., Thompson, D. M., Gulati, M., Huddleston, P., Liu, D. C., & Baroody, F. M. (2006). Improved infant swallowing after gastroesophageal reflux disease treatment: A function of improved laryngeal sensation? *The Laryngoscope, 116*(8), 1397–1403.

Verhage, C. L., Gillebaart, M., van der Veek, S. M., & Vereijken, C. M. (2018). The relation between family meals and health of infants and toddlers: A review. *Appetite, 127*, 97–109.

Weir, K., McMahon, S., Barry, L., Masters, I. B., & Chang, A. B. (2009). Clinical signs and symptoms of oropharyngeal aspiration and dysphagia in children. *European Respiratory Journal, 33*(3), 604–611.

Weir, K., McMahon, S., Barry, L., Ware, R., Masters, I. B., & Chang, A. B. (2007). Oropharyngeal aspiration and pneumonia in children. *Pediatric Pulmonology, 42*(11), 1024–1031.

Weir, K., McMahon, S., & Chang, A. B. (2005). Restriction of oral intake of water for aspiration lung disease in children. *Cochrane Database of Systematic Reviews.* https://doi.org/10.1002/14651858.CD005303.pub2

Weir, K., McMahon, S., & Chang, A. B. (2012). Restriction of oral intake of water for aspiration lung disease in children. *The Cochrane Database of Systematic Reviews.* https://doi.org/10.1002/14651858.CD005303.pub3

Wilken, M., Cremer, V., Berry, J., & Bartmann, P. (2013). Rapid home-based weaning of small children with feeding tube dependency: Positive effects on feeding behaviour without deceleration of growth. *Archives of Disease in Childhood, 98*(11), 856–861.

Williams, K. E., Field, D. G., & Seiverling, L. (2010). Food refusal in children: A review of the literature. *Research in Developmental Disabilities, 31*(3), 625–633.

Wolter, N. E., Hernandez, K., Irace, A. L., Davidson, K., Perez, J. A., Larson, K., & Rahbar, R. (2018). A systematic process for weaning children with aspiration from thickened fluids. *JAMA Otolaryngology–Head & Neck Surgery, 144*(1), 51–56.

Woods, C. W., Oliver, T., Lewis, K., & Yang, Q. (2012). Development of necrotizing enterocolitis in premature infants receiving thickened feeds using SimplyThick®. *Journal of Perinatology, 32*(2), 150–152.

Zobel-Lachiusa, J., Andrianopoulos, M. V., Mailloux, Z., & Cermak, S. A. (2015). Sensory differences and mealtime behavior in children with autism. *American Journal of Occupational Therapy, 69*(5), Article 6905185050.